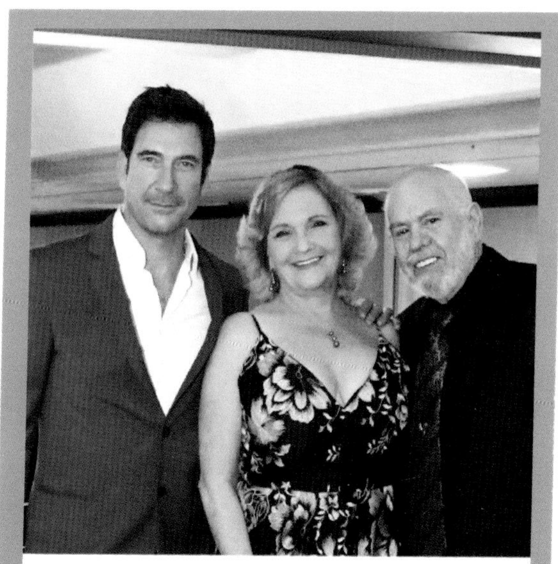

(Dylan McDermott, Je'net Kreitner, Patrick Kreitner)

"Je'net Kreitner has written a brutally honest book about surviving childhood abuse and human trafficking. It is both shocking and stunning. But the true revelation is that Je'net's heart shines bright, like a lighthouse in the deepest fog."
- Dylan McDermott

Resurrecting Hope

"No one has ever become poor by giving."

Anne Frank

"We make a living by what we get. We make a life by what we give."

Winston Churchill

"Happiness doesn't result from what we get, but from what we give."

Dr. Ben Carson

"I have found that among its other benefits, giving liberates the soul of the giver."

Maya Angelou

"It is every man's obligation to put back into the world at least the equivalent of what he takes out of it."

Albert Einstein

Resurrecting Hope

Overcoming the Invisible Violence of Child Abuse

Je'net Kreitner

Speaker House Publishing

Resurrecting Hope: Overcoming the Invisible Violence of Child Abuse

www.GrandmasHouseofHope.org

714-558-8600

Published by Speaker House Publishing

ISBN 978-1-7331249-0-4

Cover and back design by Michael de Hoyos Jr

Edited by Vern Fagan

Printed in the United States of America.

Table of Contents

Dedication

I dedicate this book to all the courageous survivors who choose to face their past and unlock a hopeful future, and to those who help them heal along the way.

Specifically, I dedicate this book to the most courageous woman I know, my daughter Jennifer, who made the brave decision to acknowledge her true spirit and beauty.

To Jeremy, who has dedicated his life in service to others with such dignity and class!

Last, but not least, I dedicate my life story to my husband, Patrick, without whom there would be no story to tell.

Special Thanks

I would like to acknowledge David Fagan for giving me the opportunity to share my story and helping me believe it was important to do so. David has the unique gift of helping others see their true potential. Thank you for sharing this gift with me and the men and women at Grandma's House of Hope. Your support made this storytelling possible.

I give special thanks to Donnie Knips. Every project needs an extraordinary organizer to bring things to fruition. So, to the Nuts and Bolts Master, I appreciate you so much! You have kept me on track and feeling optimistic.

To my writing coach, Abigail Gazda, I thank you for blessing me with your spirit, your joy, your practical wisdom, and for keeping the fire lit, even in the rain.

I must give thanks to the Staff and Board of Grandma's House, past and present. Many hands are needed to do His work. Thank you for fully showing up for the challenge each day with compassion, integrity and heart.

Thanks to all our foster and unofficially adopted children. Each moment you share with this family is a treasure. We celebrate your diversity and the common heart that beats within us.

To my biological children, Jeremy and Jennifer, I thank you for giving me permission to share as much or as little as I needed to on this journey and for the trust you showed by granting this selfless permission. It speaks truth into the silent secrecy of the past. You breathe life into me. I would be incomplete without you.

To my loving husband Patrick, thank you for showing me what unconditional love looks and feels like. All the way to the moon and back, my love.

Ultimately, I give thanks to God from whom all blessings flow. He is my source of hope, my courage and my strength. In Him all things are truly possible!

Foreword

Je'net opens her heart and soul and exposes her deepest wounds in honest and straightforward writing to reveal her journey from victim to victor. From her earliest memories of sexual abuse, to homelessness, to finding her calling and developing a charity that has provided shelter, safety, renewal, and hope for thousands of desperate people in Orange County, California, Je'net reveals the big picture of God's providence, as it's so clearly visible in her own life.

Life is the journey, not the destination. Je'net's journey uniquely equipped her to fulfill a calling that could only be accomplished with her life skill sets, acquired and honed through enduring great pain. Today we can look at her life and see the front side of a beautiful tapestry.

If your life feels like the backside of a tapestry with nothing but knots and tangles, remember that as you focus on the love that God has for you, and pass that love along to others, the topside of the tapestry will start to come into focus. All the pain and confusion, the abuse and hardship, and the failure and self-doubt will become a pathway for your fulfillment and understanding. It is never easy as evidenced in Je'net's book and life, but the road less traveled is a road that leads to spiritual abundance. Don't run away from the tough path you have been given but face it with faith. Allow God to do what he does; turn fear into action, death into life, famine into feast, and tragedy into triumph. He did it with Je'net and he will do it with you.

It is my hope that as you read this book and that you will see the active hand of God in your own life. As you read Je'net's story you will be touched and inspired.

Rev. Dr. Robert Schuller

DrSchuller.org

Introduction
A Difficult Pregnancy

I have been pregnant with this book for 60 years. It has been a heavy burden to carry. But I am confident that God has called me to share my story at this time. I know that God forgives me for all the sins that I have shared here and the actions I have taken to survive my abuse.

It has been a challenging 2-year journey of deliverance. I have felt as though I have literally been in labor, birthing this story like a midwife assisting a breach baby. The memories that crystallized during this process were re-traumatizing.

At times, I know that I have been difficult and short tempered as I walked through this minefield of memories. I pray for grace from those who were affected by this. Please forgive me and understand what a difficult road this has been to travel.

I have come to realize that it is not what happens to you in life that defines you, but how you respond to it. I understand and accept that this is the purpose God called me to in life. Suffering was part of the journey which is often required to change what needs to be changed. But the journey ends with a prize, living a life filled with God's grace and love.

My prayer is that those who know survivors will expand their hearts and minds to embrace them unconditionally and give them the time they need to heal.

"Love one another, and be kind and humble with one another. Do not pay back evil with evil or cursing with cursing; instead, pay back with a blessing, because a blessing is what God promised to give you when He called you" (1 Peter 3:8-9).

Chapter 1
Disappearing Act

It was fall and the air at night was brisk and could give you a chill all the way down to your bones. The heat in our 3-bedroom ranch house was turned up high as my mother was always concerned that my brother and I would catch a cold. I sat on my mother's bed and watched her get ready to "go on a date" with my daddy. She had carefully pressed her dress. The dress was black with sheer material at the top which gave the appearance of modesty. However, her ample bosom and cleavage were not to be tamed. Mom was a full-figured beauty with a tiny waist and oversized hips that matched her impressive bust. She had manicured short blond hair that magically seemed to stay in place. She went to the hairdressers once a week, but I could never figure out how it stayed that way until the following week's appointment. She smiled at me as she applied her red lipstick.

"One day you too will make yourself beautiful for the man of your dreams," she teased as she reached over to tickle me. I squealed and ran to see what daddy was up to.

My father, a good-looking man in the genre of "Mad Men." He was throwing away the plastic that his shirt was wrapped in from the cleaners. He was not a big man, only about 5'9", but he carried himself big. He moved over to the liquor cabinet and placed 3 ice cubes from the ice bucket into a short crystal cocktail tumbler. Aware of my presence, he tossed the tongs up in the air, caught them and acted as though he was going to tuck them in an invisible holster. Instead he pointed them at me like a gun and shot me twice. I fell to the ground in mocked agony. He laughed at my death scene and reached for me.

"Hello Princess, how's daddy's little girl?" He flashed me that irresistible smile.

I replied, "Happy daddy!" He informed me, "Carol is coming to babysit tonight!"

Daddy pulled the Canadian Scotch Whiskey out of the cabinet and poured himself a hefty 4 fingers. Taking a sip, he stretched his lips back, chuffing his pleasure.

"Carol, huh? That's great, you really like her, don't you?"

"Oh yes daddy! She lets me brush her hair and tells me stories……."

But I barely got that out because daddy was giving chase. I squealed and kept just out of his reach. Daddy managed agile calisthenics while keeping a watchful eye on his cocktail. We carried on that way until my mom and my brother Jack came to investigate the goings on. My brother, 5 years old and 2 years my senior, promptly headed directly for me. He got directly between me and my daddy and roughly pushed me down. Surprised, I landed with a thump. Triumphantly Jack looked at my dad for approval. My mom butted in, "Jack, that wasn't very nice! Help your sister up right now!"

But it was too late. I was already in tears. Jack abruptly terminated my good time. Daddy picked me up in his arms and said, "It's all right, Princess. You're okay. I am sure your brother didn't mean to do that. Did you Jack?"

Jack pouted and remained silent. My mother jumped in and promptly started to run down her worry list:

"Jerry, can you please put on your shoes? I polished them and they are right there in your closet. Are you sure you made the reservations? It's such a fancy restaurant and I would hate to be turned away."

She was starting to get worked up and both Jack and I got quiet. It was best to make yourself scarce if she was going down this path.

My father said in a soothing voice, "Dorothy calm down. I'm sure..."

At that moment, the doorbell rang, and I covered the distance to the door in a matter of seconds.

"Carol's here! Carol's here!!!"

I opened the door and there she was my most favorite baby-sitter. Tall and pretty at 16 years old. She had the most beautiful long locks I had ever seen. Carol's hair was thick, dark brown and wavy like the princess in the castle in my story book. The kind of hair I always longed for, having been short-changed with hair from my father's side of the family. My hair was thin and straight and a very uninteresting light reddish brown.

"Mr. Carman and Mrs. Carman, I am so sorry for arriving late. I was finishing up my homework and completely lost track of time. Please forgive me!"

My mom was about to share her unforgiveness, but daddy responded first.

He said, "Not to worry, Carol. We should still make it if we leave right away. Dorothy, let me help you with your coat. Doesn't my wife look lovely tonight, Carol? I'm so lucky to have married this one!" With that, he gave my mom a kiss on the lips, patted her playfully on the behind and swept her out the door.

We all watched out the big bay window in the living room, careful not to get our feet on mom's immaculate white couch. Daddy opened the door of our Chevy Impala and held my mom's hand until she was situated in the front seat. He then closed her door and glided across the front of the vehicle to settle himself in the driver's seat. They drove off and my busy 3 years old mind moved quickly on to the next possibility in front of me.

I pleaded, "Carol, Carol, can I brush your hair, please, please, pleeeeeassse?"

"Hush, Je'net, I have a surprise for all of us. Are you ready to see what it is?" Both my brother and I instantly agreed. We were ready for a surprise and looked up into her eyes with our own shiny eyes with anticipation. Carol pranced over to the door off of the kitchen porch and opened it with a "Ta-dah!"

What followed was a little awkward as there was a teenage boy on our back porch and he clearly intended to come in. The rules were no friends in the house unless mom knew about it. But he did look friendly, tall and gangly. He had a face full of freckles and a charming tilt to his nose. Carol introduced him as her boyfriend Tim. Tim smiled mischievously at us.

While rubbing my brother's head Tim said, "Hey gang, Carol asked me to teach you how to tumble. How does that sound?" Jack and I instantly liked him. With the rules forgotten, we cheered him on for our first lesson. We scrambled into the living room.

Immediately we were having the time of our lives being taught how to summersault, do the splits and finally to stand on our head! My brother, Jack, was laughing also. Jack, not as good as I was with the splits, had outdone me in a big way on the headstands. For one, he had boy pajamas on, and they were better for gymnastics than my old-fashioned floor length Lanz nightgown.

Even at 3 years old, I was modest. Mostly because my mom intentionally taught me about covering up at all times. My dresses had Peter Pan collars and were often hand made. My nightgowns covered me from head to toe. Yet, mom insisted that I not wear underwear at night after I had my bath. I remember asking her why and she said I needed to "breathe down there." I was very confused by that.

So, I was embarrassed when I did my headstand. My nightgown fell over my head and billowed to the floor. Carol and her friend could see my whole body, but I couldn't see them as my face was covered by the flowery material. I felt Tim grab my legs to help me stay balanced. Then he spread them apart and back together a few times. I didn't like that. I struggled to get my legs tucked under me and back on the ground. Everyone else was laughing but I wasn't. I felt like something wrong had just happened and ran off to my room to get "Pinkie," my little stuffed dog toy.

I was crying when Carol came in to comfort me. She told me not to be embarrassed, that we had just been playing and I should not be so sensitive. When she mentioned that she was about to make ice cream sundaes, I calmed down and managed a small smile. I tucked Pinkie under my arm and followed her into the kitchen where Jack and Tim were playing Battleship.

Shortly after ice cream, Carol tucked me into bed and read me a story from Grimm's Fairy Tales. Carol said, "I'm sorry about before, honey." She asked with a tickle, "You okay now?"

"I guess so," I replied and snuggled. "I love you Carol. Will you read me another story?"

"I love you too little one", she whispered. I fell asleep to the sound of her voice and my ballerina jewelry box playing the tune, "Around the world in 80 days."

I woke up with a start a couple of hours later. I felt confused and alarmed all at once. Tim was on my bed crouched between my knees. Once again, my stomach was cold as my nightgown was covering my face. I could still see Tim though the lace. He had a flashlight and he seemed interested in something between my legs. I felt his fingers touching me and sleepily mumbled, "Mommy…? Mommy….?" I pressed my thighs together and started to pull the nightgown off my face. Tim stood up abruptly. He stuttered when he spoke.

He stammered, "Hey kid, I was just checking in on you. I thought you were sleeping." I started to sit up, but Tim came very close to me and whispered in my ear, "I think you were having a bad dream, don't worry about it. I'll tell Carol. Go back to sleep now. Everything's ok." And with that he was out of my room closing the door quietly behind him.

A few minutes later I heard the front door open. I looked out the window and saw Tim and Carol talking on the porch. Carol put her hand tenderly on his cheek and then gave him a kiss on the lips. She headed back to the front door and I crept deep under the covers and pretended to be asleep when she poked her head in my bedroom door.

She asked, "You ok, pumpkin?"

I remained silent. I wanted to tell Carol what had happened, but I thought she might tell me I was being sensitive again and I didn't want to hear her say that.

The next day, when I woke up, I found my mom and did what you would hope your 3-year old daughter would do if something like this happened to her.

I told.

I told my mom knowing she would tell my dad. I told knowing that they would protect me. That they would believe me and make sure that Carol's friend never came back.

That evening when my daddy came home from work, my mom was waiting for him at the door with his Scotch and soda. She led him into the bedroom, and they were in there quite a while. I heard my dad raise his voice.

"That little……I can't believe Carol would let this happen. You need to talk to her, Dorothy. This happened on your watch. And get that bastard over here! I want to talk to him! TONIGHT!!"

I heard my mother crying, "I'm sorry Jerry…Jerry, please…." I went to my room and tried not to think about what they were talking about. A while later, I heard my father come out of the bedroom and head to the living room. My mother followed him and fussed with bottles at the liquor cabinet. I heard ice cubes tinkling into glasses. They were silent.

Having been summoned, Tim came over to the house a short time later. I imagine my mother requested his presence. My father responded when the doorbell rang and stepped out onto the porch. I snuck out of my room. When I didn't see my mom, I stepped closer to the door to listen. The conversation was muffled, but my father's tone was stern, and Tim's responses were timid and apologetic. It didn't last long. Tim left the porch and my dad stood there watching him leave.

My mom came up behind me and exclaimed, "Je'net! What are you doing out here? Get to bed and go on now!" She shooed me down the hallway. Jack stuck his head out the door of his room where he had been building things with his Lincoln Logs.

He questioned, "What's going on?"

"Nothing for you to worry about," mom said. "Clean up your toys and get ready for bed!"

Jack started to negotiate for more playtime, but my mom's expression shut him down and he went quickly back to his room.

Mom ushered me to the bathroom to brush my teeth. While brushing my teeth my father bellowed, "Dorothy! I need a drink!" My mom rushed me through my routine and shooed me into my room, promising to come back later and read me a story. Once again, I heard the ritual sounds of bartending.

My mom never returned as promised. I tried to wait up for her and was about to go in search of my good night kisses when daddy walked into my bedroom. I remember him standing in the doorway silhouetted by the light from the hallway. He said softly, "Je'net, I want you to show me what Tim did to you." He came in and shut the door behind him.

I did as I was told. I told him about the flashlight and showed him where I had been touched.

My daddy said, "you mean, like this...?"

I felt a chill go through my body. I couldn't process what was happening to me. I couldn't seem to speak. I felt like I was floating up above myself. I could see what was going on, but it didn't connect. His touch made me feel very confused. It felt wrong and good all at the same time. I loved my daddy. Why was he doing this?

It was all too much for me and I stopped processing what was going on. I felt some part of myself slipping away. When would he stop?

Soon there was nothing left in my heart. I thought it may have stopped beating as I had stopped breathing. I only heard his breath get heavy and fast.

"My little princess," he said. And then it was silent.

I left myself and watched from a distance. He adjusted himself and stood up. He pulled my nightgown back down and kissed me on the forehead. His eyes were not twinkling like they usually did. His expression was blank.

He just said, "Goodnight, Princess."

He closed the door and I was left alone in my darkened room. I stared into space for a while. And then I turned over on my side, pulled my knees up to my chest, hugging them close. I was sad but I had no tears. I closed my eyes and quietly disappeared.

Chapter 2
Tea Party

The next 11 years of my life are very hard to recall. I know that the abuse continued and that somewhere along the way my brother began to molest me as well. I don't know if that is because my father was abusing him also, or if he just witnessed the abuse and thought it would be ok for him to touch me the way that my father did. It's hard to pinpoint exactly when he started to abuse me, but I later recalled inappropriate episodes when we were little. These episodes happened in the car on the way back from visiting friends and relatives as early as 4 or 5 years old. It could be that I was just touching myself because I had learned that it felt good and that I comforted myself that way. Or that he was touching himself under the blankets in the back seat of the car as well. The only true specific memories I have of him intentionally sexually abusing me took place much later when I was between 11 to 16 years old before and after my father's death.

It was all so screwed up living that way.

When abuse starts that young and you live with it virtually as an everyday occurrence, it is hard to know what it right and appropriate and what isn't. I imagine that I acted in a way that made my mother uncomfortable but that she was not willing or able to see it for what it was. Years later I came to believe that my mother had also been abused as a child. Perhaps it was just too painful to face what might be happening in her own home. The culture of silence and secrecy around incest when she was growing up in the 1920's and 1930's may have led her to believe that this was an unhappy normal. Many years later she would tell me that she had no idea this was happening in her home, but the abuse was so excessive that this is hard to believe. I think she turned a blind eye to it because she felt intimidated and sensed her position with my father was being threatened. And she adored him. He was her everything.

I was often upset and tearful as a child. I would cry over the smallest of things. It didn't help that my brother seemed to really enjoy the sport of teasing me. Once when I was about 8 years old, Jack and a friend lay in wait in my bedroom while I took a shower. When I returned to my bedroom and dropped my towel, they jumped up from behind my bed and laughed at my tears of humiliation. Perhaps he thought it would be a harmless prank, but I cried for hours. Jack could be so mean. My dad would tell me not to be "such a pill." My mother repeatedly told me not to be "so super sensitive." I didn't feel like anyone was on *my* side or that they would protect me from harm.

I learned to make as little noise as possible.

When I was about 5 or 6 years old, my father was supposed to take me to a Father and Daughter Tea. My short hair was combed in a perfect pageboy with a ribbon on the side. I was wearing a light blue short dress with crisscross stitching over my chest and lots of starched taffeta. I wore bright white bobby sox with a little blue ribbon on the side and black patent leather shoes that were my favorite. I was very excited about going "on a date" with my daddy and had my stuffed toy puppy "Pinky" with me for the outing.

We were in the car a long time. Daddy gave me a sippy cup of juice and I began to feel sleepy. I uttered the well-used taunt, "Are we there yet Daddy?" Then I closed my eyes and napped peacefully until we arrived.

Instead of taking me to the Tea, my father drove me to a remote location. I don't remember the outside at all, but I remember a long wooden table with a curtain hung on a string down the middle. I was placed on the table with the curtain hitting me at my waist so that I could not see what was going on below. I was still fuzzy from my nap and couldn't sit up. There were other people there, other men besides my father. I couldn't see them but some of them touched me down there where my father did. But they were rough, not gentle like my daddy. It was strangely hushed and quiet. I only heard polaroid cameras, the electronic click and buzz as a picture would be taken, and the elongated chug when the picture would be ejected so it would develop. It sounded like a door creaking open. I knew my father was there somewhere, but he didn't answer me when I called out for him. I still felt light-headed. A male voice told me to hush or something worse would happen. He threatened to "put it inside me." I didn't know what "it" was. That scared me and only made me want to cry more but I held my breath and closed my eyes. I fought against the creeping sensation of pleasure that so deeply confused me. My pretty dress was up over my face. I mewed softly but no one comforted me. I held on tight to Pinky and felt myself drift away. I can't remember how long that went on or how it finally ended.

If we made it to the real Tea Party, I have no memories of it. I imagine we attended for a short time so that I could answer my mother's questions when we returned home. My father stopped and bought me an ice cream from the Thrifty's on the way home and told me that "Daddy's Club" was our little secret and that he was so proud of me for being such a good girl, such a little princess. He even let me have a second scoop. Chocolate chip and rocky road.

In every sense of the word, this was Human Trafficking before there was a name for it. Against my will, and at an age I could not defend myself, I was passed around for the sexual gratification of strangers. I don't know if my father benefited financially in any way for this or if it was an underground pornography-pedophile group he belonged to. My father spent time in the Philippines when he was in the Military. I suspect he brought home some very dark habits and had unlocked some raw base desires. I know that he had purchased a treehouse while he was stationed there and lived off base. He had a large trunk in the garage of our home that held his military souvenirs, but he kept it locked all the time. This trunk disappeared years later and was never recovered.

When abuse starts that young, it is hard to know what is normal and appropriate and what isn't. There were days that we were just like normal families. I was a Campfire Girl and my brother was a Boy Scout. My mother was very active in the PTA. There were birthday parties every year. We took art and music lessons just like other kids in our middle-class neighborhoods. On the surface, we looked like a happy, engaged and prosperous family.

But when the doors were locked for the night, and the window shades were drawn, a generational dark spirit lurked in every corner.

Chapter 3
Shipwrecked

My father loved the open sea and we owned several medium sized sailboats before we made the long distance move from California to Ohio in 1967. My mother didn't like to sail (it got her hair all messed up) so it was usually just some configuration of my dad, my brother and me. I loved the feeling of the wind in my hair and sitting at the bow of the boat. My father would buy me a 5-cent bag of sunflower seeds when we stopped at the liquor store to buy his beer. I spent hours sucking on the salty shells. My brother would get sweet tarts and sometimes share them with me. I was responsible for untying the rope that bound us to the pier. Jack was given the more important duties. Once we set off, my job was mostly to stay out of the way. There was a galley below with cushions that formed a bed and fishnet hammocks that held important provisions. I would be asked to straighten up the galley, but I didn't like "going below" because my dad would always follow me down the steep stairs to "give me a hand."

It would seem like I would have tried to avoid my father at all costs, but the fact of the matter was, I worshiped him. While my mother would distance herself from me, and my brother would antagonize me, my dad would be the one I would run to when I got my feelings hurt (which was often) or scraped a knee. The good memories I have with my daddy were creative times. He played folk guitar and entertained at lots of barbeques and when friends came over to visit.

I used to sit next to him and sing and loved the attention that I got for having a strong and pleasant voice. People were always surprised and commented on how such a big voice came out of such a small child. I soon learned to harmonize but my mother didn't like that because she couldn't hold a melody unless everyone else was singing the same part. We would laugh and poke fun at her. She soon started to excuse herself from the music circles and instead would clean up in the kitchen or talk to the other wives. Another degree of separation.

Daddy was adventurous and quite artistic. One day a baby grand piano showed up to take center stage in our living room. He was gifted and taught himself to play classical piano by ear. Not long after, he decided he would start painting. He set up an easel and oil paints in the basement. He completed some very nice pieces. One that he loved the most was of a man fishing on a pier with three very young girls. It appears to be set in the Philippines, and everyone is in shadows. This painting occupied prime real estate on the family room wall for many years. I still have this painting but cannot bring myself to display it.

I took after his creative side and loved to be the center of attention. This led me in later years to seek professional training in both music and theater. My brother Jack had talent as well and inherited my father's love for jazz. Jack tried several wind instruments before he settled on the saxophone. Yet, it was easier to learn to sing than learn an instrument, so I got most of the attention for years. I think this bothered him when he was younger. Later, he became quite the professional, even touring with Frank Zappa and opening for B.B. King in the late 1980's. It appeared that both of us were reaching out to the world, rather than to our own family for acceptance and love.

We moved multiple times while I was a child. Four times by the time I was 10. Every location a nice home, each one a little better than the last. The third home in Playa del Rey was near the marina where our boat was docked. Mom and Dad designed the house themselves and hired construction contractors to complete the plans. It was a lovely 2 story 4-bedroom home with a formal dining room, living room and family room. My mom envisioned the back yard with a pretty fountain and lots of concrete, not terribly kid friendly for an 8 and 10-year old. We each had our own room and used the fourth bedroom as a playroom, complete with bumper pool and our own turntable for the latest new sounds of the Monkeys and the Beatles.

My mother loved this home and took great care with it. For the first time we had a maid. Betsy helped with the housekeeping, but I still remember my mom doing a lot of the heavy work. She was a bit obsessive about it. *Everything* had to be ironed including bed sheets, undershirts, even underwear and socks! There could be no dust anywhere! Her friends used to joke that they would never pop in on Dorothy and find anything out of place. I believe this was where my mother had permission to be in complete control and she was almost desperately compulsive about it. If there was one thing she truly excelled at, it was creating the illusion that our family was just like an episode of "Father Knows Best" or "Leave it to Beaver." Everything had to look perfect on the outside to make up for what was going on inside.

There was a lot of upheaval about our last move together as a family. I remember it being explained that my father had an excellent opportunity to "climb the ladder" at Parker Hannifin Aerospace. He would be a Vice President with a salary of $40,000, a substantial amount in 1967 when the average salary was circling around $19,000. He would have a fancy office all to himself and many people would report to him.

My mother absolutely did not want to go and let my father know it at every opportunity. She had her dream house and all her friends. Why should they move from California to Ohio? She cried and cried and complained. My dad would talk about how he looked forward to exposing his family to all four seasons. When Jack and I heard there would be snow a lot of our complaints went away. I would very much miss my best friend Karin, but ultimately my father always made the final decisions. He left for Ohio on his own to purchase a house and start anew.

I often wonder if there was something just a little more intentional about the whole reassignment. There was urgency about the whole thing that felt unnatural, as though it were the solution to a problem. We had built the last home with an expectation of staying in Playa Del Rey a good long time. Were people getting suspicious?

Chapter 4
Coming of Age

The house in Ohio was large and spacious, but only had 3 bedrooms. To my mother it was a step down. No house could hold a candle to her dream home back in Playa del Rey. The kitchen was large but old fashioned instead of the modern one she had loved. There was a breakfast nook in the kitchen where we would eat all family meals. At the rear entrance there was a back porch/mudroom with a laundry and a half bath. Also, the house had a formal dining room, a living room, and a den which we used as a family room. There was a screened-in patio that looked out over our 1 ½ acres of forest. We were at the top of a hill and our back yard was the neighborhood's favorite spot for winter sledding before and after we arrived. This was a big advantage for making friends. There was one average sized bedroom downstairs next to a full bath that would also serve as a guest bathroom and two other bedrooms upstairs. After much discussion, my parents took the downstairs room and delegated the upstairs for the kids.

The upstairs of the house was unfairly divided into two bedrooms with a shared bath. One bedroom was very large. It had over 550 square feet with a library workspace as well as an area for a table with 4 chairs. Additionally, it was adjacent to a finished attic space that was accessible only through that room. It was definitely prime real estate. I was awarded this room to the great dismay and protests of my older brother who should have by rights gotten it. In my upstairs bedroom there was enough room for a King size bed, so I inherited my parent's old one. My parents downsized to a Queen, the largest the downstairs room could manage comfortably. My room was easily the most spacious and nicest room in the house. It was also the farthest away from my parent's room below. Jack was assigned the smallest bedroom with enough space for only a twin bed. There were protests from both my brother and my mom, who said Jack was the oldest and should have the larger room, but my dad stood firm that his little Princess would inherit this prestigious space and so it was mine (and his).

Off the kitchen there was a door and flight of stairs that led to a large basement. The basement was finished on one side as a game room where the bumper pool table was re-established. It also sported a bar with bar stools. We thought they were so cool! On the opposite end of the recreation room was a set of couches. A great place for tweens to hang out! Through another door was an unfinished space just as big with a large worktable with all kinds of tools and gadgets. It was here in the basement that my father would hide his cigarettes by the furnace. He had promised to quit once we moved. Also, in this part of the basement he would paint with vigor and tinker with his other love, photography. He was always splicing film together down there, for hours at a time.

The basement would also become the home for all my whiskered pets such as gerbils, hamsters and mice. I had more than 75 of them! I had started with just 2 pet mice and subsequently added the other creatures. Before long they had multiplied several times over. I would take full litters of the bald squirming newborns over to my friend Helen's house. Before long, our mothers realized what we were doing and took most of them out to the woods behind the house and set them free.

Life in Ohio started out rough for me. I had made a good neighborhood friend over the summer with Helen who lived down the street. Yet, she did not stand by me when school started, and important alliances were forged between her and the cool kids. It was a small town called Pepper Pike and new families were rare. There was a buzz about the family from California and expectations that we might be like the popular Disney icons, Annette Funicello and Frankie Avalon. Beach

Blanket Bingo was a very hot movie at that time with many parents forbidding their children to watch the indecent teenage love story. I just did not fill that movie star bill. I was still round with baby fat and my mother dressed me in a manner she thought was conservative and 1960's Baptist appropriate. Her rules about the length of my skirts, the modest necklines, not to mention a bad bowl haircut brought out the bully in the popular kids. I really struggled in middle school.

I was a very unhappy kid and needy for any attention I could get at home as school was so unwelcoming. Unfortunately, that only drew me closer to my dad. In his way he would reassure me that I was beautiful and talented.

My parents paid for voice lessons and I joined the choir, where I would effortlessly land solos and get some needed positive feedback. I spent most of my free time reading books and writing long letters to my friend Karin back home and to my great grandmother.

I started to learn French at school and the letters to and from my great grandmother were always written in this romantic language. She was fluent and would send my letters back to me with her corrections. She was mysterious, eccentric and brilliant. I loved her. I had never met my great grandfather as he had died many years before I was born, but when we visited her, I always thought it was so exotic that she lived in a high-rise apartment building. It was a small place, and everything was just so. She had a collection of small ceramic animals, mostly dogs, displayed on nearly every surface. I still have some of them. I have a very fond memory of making holiday fudge with her one afternoon. She let me get the kitchen very messy and didn't seem to mind. I later came to find out that she had opened the very first day care center for working moms in the 1930's and was an avid women's rights advocate. She passed away at 98 years old while we were living in Ohio. Only my father returned for the funeral. It broke my heart not to say goodbye.

Things improved by the time I reached my freshman year in high school. I had been noticed for my singing abilities in 8th grade and was recommended by my teachers for the high school choir and drama club. At 5'4", I had slimmed down to a trim 105 pounds. My hair had grown out to shoulder length in a current page boy style. Before long I had found a niche and even landed a spot in the Broadway Review opposite the most popular and handsome senior boy. I performed a tap dance and sang, "I want to be Happy." I then landed the role of Mariel in "Ah Wilderness" and was on my own little road to fame and happiness. I hung out with "bandies" and learned to twirl a baton and a flag with other girls who supported the Marching Band. We wore short red skirts that my mother had no control over and were so proud of our Nancy Sinatra white "walking" boots. The band enjoyed hanging out with the flag twirlers and socializing at our after-game parties. We were all a step down from the Football players and cheerleaders, but we thought we were special. Soon the Pepper Pike Polka Party Partners Club was formed. Yes, we polka-ed… and it was cool.

I was now 14 years old and was well liked in my circle. Life was getting better, so I thought. I successfully suppressed all of what was transpiring with my dad (and now my brother) and woke up to a new day every morning with no memory of any horror that had taken place the night before. I had come to a point where I could fool even myself.

I started my period after most of my friends. They were always talking about "having their friend visit" but I was embarrassed and could not comment. I may have even lied about having mine. Girls were starting to use tampons instead of their mothers old fashioned pads. I tried to practice using them but could not manage. I would get anxious and nervous, but I didn't know why. It would always bring me to tears. Perhaps it triggered the memories from the Tea Party when I was threatened with penetration to keep me quiet. When my mother had told me about menstruation at 10 years old, I was terrified and could not stop crying. But when it finally happened early in my fourteenth year, I was glad because I wouldn't have to pretend in gym class anymore. I told my mom in confidence that I had started to bleed and assumed she would keep it between us. But she told my dad in front of me even though I begged her not to tell.

I remember him saying to me, "So I guess today you became a woman." It was an extremely awkward moment. I sensed a sadness from him and that made me incredibly uncomfortable. Later, I came downstairs dressed for my first Homecoming dance. I wore a very short cream-colored dress with my first pair of nylons and high heels. He got up off the couch and made a circle around me unsteadily. With his speech a little slurred by the Scotch, he commented proudly, "Look Dorothy the girls got legs!" Neither one of us laughed. I felt my face go red and turned away.

Summer came. My brother Jack had begun performing with "Up with People," a live musical review with upbeat patriotic themes. There were singers, dancers and a full orchestra. Jack had auditioned at 16 and landed a spot in the touring company playing his beloved saxophone. After rehearsing all spring, the group was set for a summer tour. It was a big deal for my mom to let him go. She was always extremely protective of us both. We had earlier curfews and less telephone time than virtually all our friends. Jack would be gone for three weeks! Sending him off was a tearful event but my father totally supported Jack being able to go, even though it meant him being gone for Father's Day that year.

Around this time, my dad had started to have some health issues. It seemed he was always complaining of heartburn. Evening found him alternating his Scotch with Maalox or milk from the refrigerator. I knew he was smoking again although he had tried to quit several times. The cigarette butts in the basement furnace were piling up high and smoked down to the very end. He smelled like smoke but tried to hide it with Old Spice cologne. He broke out in a sweat and became short of breath, taking several breaks when he went out to do the yard work he loved.

During this time, I remember he started to ask me to take a bath in the downstairs bathroom when my mom was out at the store. We were alone in the house several times after Jack left on tour. After I got in the tub, he would come in, undress and shower in the same bathroom where he could see me through the shower glass. I knew what he was doing. He would ask me to get clean under the faucet and watch me as the water flowed over my body. He would step out of the shower completely naked and dry off in front of me. I knew what could happen if he had sex with me now that I was menstruating. I became especially fearful and avoided him. For this first time in my life, I started to hate him a little.

Chapter 5
Father's Day

It was the night before Father's Day. Dad had made several trips to the fridge for a milk fix and was chewing on Rolaids like they were popcorn. He didn't eat much at dinner and excused himself for bed early. I have a very vivid memory of my mom telling me to go into their bedroom to wish him a happy Father's Day and kiss him good night. I refused. My mom was surprised. I usually did what I was told. She changed her tone from a request to a demand. I walked into their bedroom and dad was in bed propped up with pillows.

I said, "Good night daddy, hap……." But I couldn't finish the salutation. I stood there on the far side of the room and fidgeted. He looked at me with a funny expression on his face. I couldn't read it. It was all at once hurt and apologetic and scared. I averted my eyes and said, "good night" again and went upstairs to my own bed. It was weird sleeping upstairs all alone with Jack away on tour. And my father's demeanor had shaken me. But I had become an expert at turning off my feelings, so I closed my eyes and soon went to sleep.

I awoke with a start. I heard my mother screaming my father's name

"Jerry!! Jerry!!! Oh my God, Jerry!"

I scrambled from my bed and made my way downstairs. It was at dawn. The sun was only just beginning to light the horizon. When I entered the bedroom all the lights were on and my mother was struggling with my father who appeared to be gasping for air. His face was bright red and his eyes were bulging open and terrified. He couldn't seem to catch a breath. Through her panic, Mom managed to communicate that I should go to her side. She told me to hold him up so he could breathe. I did as I was told, frightened with his heaving body and gasping breaths. My mother left the room to use the kitchen telephone to call 911. I could hear her screaming on the phone for help, for someone to come quickly. Dad grabbed me by my nightgown desperately with one hand, searching my face and reaching out in a panic. He was starting to turn purple and trying to grab his chest with his free hand.

Thankfully, my mother returned and took him from me. She directed me to ride my bike down the hill to the neighbor's house. The one where the doctor lived. I was unsure where that was, but she said it was near her friend, Mrs. Bailey's house. I had done some babysitting for this family on occasion, so I got my bearings and took off on my bike down the long hill of our street. About ½ mile down, I stopped at Mrs. Bailey's house and pounded on the door, but no one answered. I then began to frantically knock on every door on the street. Finally, someone came out to all the ruckus I was causing and pointed to the doctor's front door. I laid into that door yelling, "My dad is dying, my dad is dying!! You have to come help! Help me, please help me!!!"

Finally, the doctor's wife answered the door and told me her husband would be right out. She said, "Wait here and we'll give you a ride back up the street as soon as the doctor is dressed." But I couldn't just stand there doing nothing. I was frantic to get back to my dad.

I ditched my bike and ran up the back way through the woods behind the houses on Belgrave Road. It was a long uphill climb and I was hysterical. I tripped and fell several times twisting my ankle and noticing for the first time that I was barefoot. By the time I emerged from the trees the paramedics were loading my dad in an ambulance. I waved hysterically for them to wait but they ignored me. They packed him into the back of the vehicle and slammed the doors before I could get to them. I stared frozen to the spot as they raced off to the hospital. My mom looked pale and lost.

She told me to put some clothes on so we could follow.

I don't remember how we got to the hospital. My mom was in no shape to drive. It might have been the doctor from down the hill or Mrs. Bailey. I do remember the waiting room and sitting all alone on a hard-plastic chair as my mother paced back and forth. She never looked at me or talked to me or comforted me. There were other people there for various reasons and for their own loved ones, but it was like no one could see me. When the hospital doctor came out after what seemed such a long time, he talked quietly to my mom alone in the corner of the waiting room. She let out a low moan that got louder and louder and then started to yell and punch him. Nurses ran quickly to his aid prying my mom away from him. It took a few people to restrain her. Finally, someone came with a needle and gave her a shot which knocked her out. From then on, she was in a daze. I stood up tentatively, wondering if I should go to her, but she frightened me and so I sat back down and stared at the goings on from my chair. It was as if no one I knew was there. No one came over to comfort me. I was alone. I didn't belong. I was invisible to everyone who bustled through the room.

I have virtually no recollection of leaving the hospital or how we got home. But suddenly we were there, and it was just my mom and me. She cried. I was silent. She would look right through me and say, "What am I going to do? How am I going to tell Jack?" She seemed to be concerned about my brother but oblivious that I was right there in front of her. I just looked at her and tried to be small. She cried and cried and cried. I thought it would never end.

Neighbors started to arrive at the front door with food. I thought that was strange because everyone had always used the back door off the driveway before that. The only people who ever came to the front door were my dad's business friends. And those people were not here. There was so much food. It was everywhere on every surface of the kitchen and dining room. And everyone was trying to feed me and my mom. She refused every bite, barely drinking a glass of water. The neighbors focused on me then, offering me plate after plate. I reacted differently. The food seemed to sooth me and I ate slowly but deliberately through every offering. My mother had still not spoken directly to me or comforted me. But now I finally got her attention. Her first words to me after my dad died were, "How can you eat at a time like this? Don't you care that your father is dead?" You may wonder how eating disorders begin. This is a classic example of the power that words can have over children. That was the beginning of a long history of eating disorders.

Somehow the decision was made not to tell my brother about dad's death until he came home from tour, which was only a day or two later. I remember there was discussion about how hard it would be for him to manage the rest of the bus trip if he knew. I observed internally that my mom was taking care of him even when he wasn't there but still had not paused to check in with me.

By that time my mother's best friend, Elaine, had arrived from California. She was constantly by her side. Elaine was a matter of fact pleasant woman with a sense of humor but not particularly affectionate. I remember thinking for many years that she didn't like me, but I think that was just her way. My mother had always referred to her as her best friend. Much later I asked Elaine about their close relationship. She told me that they really were not that close and didn't spend that much time together. To her credit, she really showed up for mom in her time of need. She was practical, had an agenda, and walked my mom through the next steps in the following week. I don't know how my mom would have managed without her.

Jack walked through the back door. The smile on his face evaporated as my mother rushed to him and embraced him as though she could never let go. I remember thinking how odd it was she had none of this compassion or empathy for me. He was taken to my mom's bedroom where my mom broke the news. When they emerged, his eyes were puffy and red, and he wouldn't look anyone in the eye. My mom cried. He cried. I could not cry. I had spent so many years holding back my tears and masking how I truly felt inside, I just didn't know how to let it go.

Was I thinking, "Is it finally over?"

Finding the corner of the room, I watched in silence. People were unnerved by me and kept a distance.

A memorial happened. My father's body was not there. It had been cremated. I didn't know most of the people who attended. I don't remember if any family members from California were there. I think that if they had been, they would have stayed with us, and they did not. Elaine stayed. I remember sitting in the front pew of a church we had never attended. I listened to a man talk about my father knowing he had never met him. No one else spoke. It seemed to be over quickly. After the funeral we ate the last big buffet of food. I sat on the staircase and ate. No one told me I couldn't eat there even though I knew it was forbidden to eat anywhere but at the kitchen table. I watched an endless stream of people. Most of them came from my father's workplace. They approached my mother and held her hands for a moment before they walked away and back to their counterparts. Unlike any other gathering at the house, no one smiled or laughed. The women gathered in the kitchen and talked in low voices and they glanced at my mom from time to time. My mom stayed separated and sat on the living room couch as people paused briefly to speak with her.

Then……nothing. People went home, went back to their two parent households, back to their lives, back to work, and back to school. Elaine went back to California. But nothing was ever the same for us.

When I went back to school that fall, schoolmates didn't know how to deal with me. Should they acknowledge they knew my dad was dead and that I was essentially half an orphan? Would they say the wrong thing and upset me? I watched my mother's friends leave her one by one. She was no longer asked to lunch with the other moms. There was a sense that a widowed woman would be a threat to their husbands. My mother became exceedingly depressed. Later she would tell me that she would get Jack and me up for school, make our lunches, get us on the bus, and then go back to bed until just before we would arrive home from school. She became quite dependent on valium, the most prescribed drug in the US between 1969 and 1982 for treating anxiety and panic attacks. Later she would threaten to commit suicide with these same pills.

As distant as my mother was with me, she pressured me to sleep with her every night in her bedroom, in the bed she had shared with my dad. At first, I was grateful for the attention. She would sometimes scratch my back or ask me to scratch hers. We would try and talk to each other. She would occasionally ask me about my day, but she never had anything to say about hers. And, almost every night she ended up crying. If I tried to console her by snuggling close, she would just get worse. Ultimately, I would try and get as far away from her as I could, hugging my side of the bed, pulling the pillow around my head to drown out her sobs. I never had permission to cry myself because I knew it would make her cry too, so I just kept holding it all in. And because I didn't cry, she accused me of not caring. After a summer of this, I asked to go back to my bedroom upstairs. The look on her face broke me down and I continued to sleep down there for over a year. We made plans to go back to California as soon as my brother graduated high school in 1973.

Chapter 6
Dark Poetry

After my father passed, we stayed in Ohio through the end of the school year so my brother could graduate high school with his peers. Then we returned to California. My mother rented a house in Irvine. Jack attended school at Saddleback College. I enrolled at University High for my junior and senior year. During those 2 years my mother worked hard at holding things together when my brother was around, but felt very free to share her grief, anger and desperation in front of me when he wasn't. She would miraculously recover from a screaming match with me the moment Jack walked in the door after his college classes. I would remain wild eyed and hyperventilating, still caught up in my mom's hysteria. That's all my brother would see – Je'net going off again.

Jack had begun to make late night visits into my room after mom was tucked away with Scotch and her pills. The abuse mimicked what I had experienced with my father except it was completely void of emotion or any pretense of affection. It seemed that wherever I turned, I became the brunt of the battle and the lamb brought to slaughter. By this time my brother was nearing 18 years old and had to know that his behavior with me was inappropriate. For that matter, why did I not feel that I could rebuke him? Why did I let that keep happening? I would usually just pretend to be asleep, like I had for years with my father. As a female I was brought up to accept that I had a role to be submissive. To be used for someone else's pleasure, literally without any other value. We never discussed it out loud and the topic was so taboo. Could it be that both of us thought this was just the way families behaved?

There were several times my mother would tell me that she had enough pills to finish her off and that maybe that's just what she should do. I would try and tell her that life was still worth living and that she couldn't do that to Jack. The absence of her worrying about what it would do to me was palpable. I was the one she came to when she needed to vent and be heard, but he was the one she worried about. It seemed to matter to her very much what Jack thought of her, but that didn't seem to apply to me. She was very unstable and did not seek mental health support. She just kept refilling the anti-anxiety prescriptions from the doctor.

Once again, she threatened to kill herself with pills. She tore out of the driveway in the family car screeching the tires when she hit the asphalt. I was terrified she would get in a wreck and kill herself or someone else! I called Elaine in a panic asking for advice. Elaine told me I should call the police and that she would head over to the house. About 45 minutes later my mom re-appeared, red eyed and walking unsteadily. She avoided my gaze and went silently to her room and locked the door.

When Elaine arrived, my mom played it down entirely. The police were stopped before they could arrive because mom didn't want to alarm Jack. After Elaine left my mom lit into me for calling her. I had embarrassed her with one of her few remaining friends. How could I do such a thing? It never occurred to her that I loved her enough to try and save her life.

In my senior year mom downsized and bought a condo. She preferred the concept of a Homeowner's Association that would take care of the landscaping, something my father had always done. Maybe she thought she might meet someone. After we moved to the condo things did not get any better. In fact, they got worse. I was spending more time with my high school friends and stayed away from the house as much as I could. My mom started to call me a whore and believed that I was sleeping around.

In fact, I had become infatuated with a student professor from UCI. He came to our high school to teach an Advanced Poetry class to the English Honor students. I lied to my mom about spending the night with a friend and set up a rendezvous on the beach in Newport. He was very mysterious and exotic to me. I swooned when he read me his raw and esoteric poetry. He kissed me tenderly under the light of a full moon. When he invited me back to his apartment, I went willingly. Yet, when we were alone things got physical very quickly and I began to panic. This was the first time I was engaging in sexual activity with anyone other than my father or brother. I started to head for the door, but he got between me and the exit. Although I said "no" and pleaded with him to stop, he insisted he found me irresistible and forced himself on me. I went numb and waited for it to end. When it was over, I was in tears. He was confused and a bit angry with me for "leading him on." I shot out of there and walked all the way back to my friend's house where I was supposed to be spending the night. I had been raped but I didn't see it that way. I had come to accept the role of victim. This is just what happened to me. I never told anyone about what happened that night until I was nearly 30 years old.

After the rape, I went through a period of depression and emotional outbursts that led my mother to finally seek help for me. She tried to convince me I was having trouble coping with my father's death. I saw my first psychologist, Mr.

Stevens, at age 16. He worked out of his beautiful beachside home in Laguna. He made me tea and was kind and patient. It didn't take him long to start asking questions about my childhood. He asked me to share a lot about my dad. I didn't know the answers to any of the questions he asked me about my childhood because I had blocked them. My mom kept after him to talk to her after my sessions, but he said he needed more time with me. The questions got more and more personal. After seeing him for about 6 weeks, he did meet with my mom before my scheduled session. I didn't see him that day or any day after. My mom emerged from his house breathless and ordered me into the car. She was red faced and crying. I was disappointed because I had liked this man. I felt safe with him and I was starting to trust him. I will never know what he said to my mom, but I imagine he tried to tell her that something inappropriate had gone on between my dad and me. I think he was getting close to the truth and my mom did what she had done all my life. She closed the door and looked the other way.

Chapter 7
All the World is a Stage

I had wholeheartedly jumped into drama and chorus and madrigal singers at Uni High. I was cast in several roles including Golde in Fiddler on the Roof, Louisa in The Fantasticks, Mrs. Noah in the opera, Noah's Fludde, and others. Upon graduation I took home many awards, including Best Actress, Best Supporting Actress, and The National Choral Award. I sang in the Honor Choir and nailed the soprano solo, the only alto brave enough to audition. I graduated with decent grades and was accepted at CSU Fullerton on an Opera Scholarship. I was still 17 years old but entirely ready for the emancipation I believed college would give me from my mom.

I went through the audition process at CSUF and was honored with a spot in the alto section of the University Singers, usually only open to college juniors and seniors. I wanted to double major in drama. I auditioned for the theatre department with a monologue from "Sybil," which is a screenplay about a victim of childhood abuse so extreme it resulted in multiple personality disorder. I remember the quiet moment when I finished the monologue and the positive comments from the judges about my performance. I was surprised to be placed in advanced acting my freshman year, skipping beginning and intermediate altogether. Then again, I had been acting since I was three years old! For my senior classmates, I seemed to have come from nowhere. A rumor got started that I was an exchange student and that I may have been previously married. What? Perhaps it was the way I carried myself, or just a way to explain why I was in these advanced classes. I can't really remember, but I played along and took college on whole heartedly. I took general education classes toward graduation. But I wanted only music, theatre and English and focused my attention there. After all, how would those other classes help me to become a famous performer? As a freshman, I was cast in 2 main stage productions, again normally reserved for upperclassmen who had already paid their dues. I was away from the oppression at home and was flourishing.

I had a particularly rewarding experience when I was a freshman. Richard Dreyfus was set to come to our campus and run an afternoon workshop. He was an A list actor with the blockbuster Jaws behind him and Close Encounters having just hit the theatres. He shared some of his insights from his acting career and then asked if anyone was working on a scene who would be willing to come forward so he could critique it. Everyone seemed to clam up, intimidated by the idea of having such a famous respected actor give them notes and direction. I paused as well but ultimately was the first to put my hand high up in the air. He asked me what I was working on? I told him, "Who's Afraid of Virginia Wolf?"

He said, "Okay, you must be playing Honey, right?" He gave me the once over; seeing a slim 5'4" big busted woman with a sweet disposition. Based on his observation of me he assumed that I would be working on the ingénue role. I said, "Actually, I am playing Martha." This was the Elizabeth Taylor role - an alcoholic wife with a tragic hidden past for which she won an Academy Award.

Richard Dreyfus looked me up and down and said, "Well, you've got guts kid. I got to give you that. What scene?"

Enthusiastically I said, "Hump the Hostess!"

This is the height of the play where all the characters have had too much to drink and all hell breaks loose. Martha and her husband, George, really go at it.

He raised his eyebrows and said, "Well, as luck would have it, I know that scene, let's give it a go."

It was magic. Something I will always remember. Amazingly, I acted this scene all the way through with Richard Dreyfus! I couldn't believe he knew every one of George's lines. Our characters were playful and coy, furious and hateful. In the end we got a standing ovation from the class. Afterward, about six of us went across the street to Hoff's Hut for fried onion rings with Richard. I found him to be a funny down to earth guy. This is probably my most memorable highlight from college.

In December of 1975, as soon as I turned 18 years old, I moved out on my own with the Social Security survivor benefits from my father. My mother began to date David Stewart, a man that she had met through business functions with my father. Many years before, David had worked at the same company as my dad. Our families had even come together for special occasions a few times over the years. David had 8 children and had lost his wife to cancer a few years before. They shared their common grief and I think my mom found his Catholic faith attractive. It had helped sustain this man with so many children to care for. About a year later they married. There were just 2 daughters left at home to raise and my mother happily stepped back into the role of wife and hostess.

Things started to get better between my mother and myself after she married. I sang at her wedding while my brother played guitar. Together we performed "The Wedding Song" by the Carpenters. She and I started speaking to each other by phone several times a week. We got along much better now that my mom had rejoined the community she understood. I had proved myself capable of living on my own, and she relaxed her grip on me.

I was excited about the new season of plays at school. This year we were going to perform Shakespeare's Antony and Cleopatra. I saw myself holding the title role. I engaged in an intimate relationship with one of my drama teachers. He was married but separated from his wife. He happened to be directing this Shakespearean play. He cast me as Charmaine, Cleopatra's handmaiden, and as understudy for the leading role. It was frowned upon to complain about getting any role in a main stage production, so I buckled down humbly to learn both roles. As fate would have it, Cleopatra contracted mononucleosis and had to back out of the play about 2 weeks from opening. I felt bad for her. She was doing a great job, but I was secretly exhilarated to take on the role as her understudy. All my hard work was to pay off! But my director/lover had different ideas. He made a controversial decision to bring in an outside professional actress to play the role – his estranged wife. So uncomfortable! Here I was, sleeping with her husband and playing her subservient handmaiden. As soon as the last curtain fell, I left college to move to LA and start my professional career. I moved in with my new lesbian girlfriend, April.

April and I had met at a cast party. She was older than me and already performing professionally at Knott's Berry Farm in the Chu Chu Lavern show. Of course, she was Chu Chu. She was a darling blond haired impish looking creature with a childlike speaking voice. She had a very impressive low alto belt that took everyone by surprise and had quite a following back in those pre-social media days. I was charmed by her and her with me. We fell in love.

We forged our way to Hollywood. We were set for the big time. We rented an apartment with a flamboyant gay man named Emilio Oliveros. We set up house there for about 6 months, living in a Hollywood where you still had to keep your private affairs private. No holding hands in public and no public display of affection. I loved this woman. She adored me. But in the end living with her made me realize that I ultimately wanted to be in relationship that would eventually include children. In those days it was unheard of for a gay couple to adopt. It was a sad breakup. She was a lesbian and I was bi-sexual and ultimately that fact caused the split in our relationship. She moved out and I got a gig with a touring musical review. The group was much like "Tony Orlando and Dawn," an American Pop music group that was popular in the

70's. We called ourselves, "Bob Gregory with Love."

We performed pop tunes and played in nightclubs from Green Bay Wisconsin to Reno Nevada. I was a backup singer with Connie, a girl from Missoula Montana. She was a statuesque gorgeous blond beauty and I was the cute spunky pixie. She played dumb and I was sarcastic, what Joyce DeWitt was to Suzanne Somers on Three's Company. We got to work up an opening act, just the two of us with the band, so we got individually showcased as well.

Bob was a Joel Grey (of "Cabaret" fame) look alike. He was adequately talented but not enough talent for the big time. But the gig paid well, and it was professional. Although we stayed in some seedy dives on the road. I had permission to take my precious sidekick Kermit the dog with me.

Kermit was a Shih Tzu-Pomeranian mix who had Gidget's disease – he was terminally cute. This little pup was in 3 plays with me and my first movie. Kermit worked as a prop. He replaced a box of bonbons by sitting on my lap in a period piece called, "The Necklace." "The Necklace" was an AFI independent film. Everyone fell in love with this pooch. He went to college with me and preceded me to all my classes and rehearsals. Kermit was smart enough to never cross the tape that outlined where the set pieces would eventually go. He had the ability to jump straight up into the air from all fours and fit nicely in my backpack. Words can't express how much this little guy meant to me. He would survive a couple of near-death experiences, including walking off the roof of a 3-story building in Utah into the snow below. Up until the very end at 17 years old and blind, he could always find his way to a piece of bacon.

Before we left on our 6-month tour, we performed in a local nightclub in North Hollywood. I remember my mother came to see the show with David and her best friend Elaine. And I remember how she cried when she saw me sing "Play that Funky Music, White Boy." Our costumes ranged from formal sexy to elevator sneakers and Fredericks of Hollywood hot pants with rainbow suspenders. Not exactly the future she had foreseen for her daughter. But I was excited to be finally performing for a living. My mother could not persuade me to reconsider, no matter how hard she pleaded with me.

Before I left on the road, I had taken a stab at auditioning for the American Conservatory Theatre in San Francisco. They had a very prestigious advanced acting program at the time and only accepted 40 to 50 students a year from across the country. My mother still hoped I would not go on the road with the band. She promised me that if I got in, she would completely support me and pay for school. When I went up to San Francisco for my audition, I got very adventurous and walked into some scary districts without knowing I could be in danger. I remember making acquaintance with a sad looking young man in the park in the downtown district. It was the season of flower children and love. The young man looked downtrodden and hungry and I befriended him with a meal at a local restaurant. I began to think I was in trouble when he started to nod out in his soup. Only then did I realize he was high as a kite on heroin. I pretended I was going to use the restroom, and hastily paid the check. He began to make a scene as I left. I felt very bad for the restaurant owner who was left to deal with him.

I went on to see the show at the Geary Theatre that night. As I remember it was a Chekov play. Then I went back to my hotel room. I was exhausted and fell asleep with my contact lenses in – a fatal mistake.

When I awoke on the morning of my audition, I could barely open my eyes. I spent several hours with a cold compress over my eyes with all the curtains drawn in the room. I could not even practice my two monologues. It was unacceptable to make excuses in an audition, so I went to the theatre full of outward confidence before the jury panel. Inside of myself I was screaming with pain from the bright lights in the room. I managed to get through both "Barefoot in the Park" and "Midsummers Night's Dream." It didn't go badly, although I had unwanted tears stream down my face at the most inappropriate moments. They must have been so confused! I thanked them for their consideration and trudged back to my room to pack and fly back home. I knew I had blown my best chance of ever being a professional stage actress and my heart was broken.

When we were on the road for about 6 weeks, I got word through my very relieved mother that I had been accepted at ACT – a miracle!! I promptly gave notice that I would be leaving at the 4-month mark of my contract which did not make my band mates or my boss very happy. In fact, when it came time to leave, the bass player tried to kidnap poor little Kermit in a misguided attempt to force me to stay. I literally had to sneak away under cover of night. My Hollywood boyfriend at the time (Mark) drove up to Reno to rescue me. We drove all night back home, having each swallowed a black beauty (some very potent speed) to keep awake.

Still a little buzzed, Mark deposited me at my mother's house in Tarzana. It was still dark, and my mom put me up in the guest room. I couldn't sleep. I unwisely decided to give my bangs a trim. Several hours later most of my hair was in the sink as I kept snipping away to make things even. It was a mess. My mom had to take me to a hairdresser the next day to try and salvage what was left. I arrived at ACT with a decidedly butch little curly haircut. Yes, I was so embarrassed, but tremendously excited!!

I thoroughly adored San Francisco and all the energy of Haight Ashbury during the celebratory hippy era. School was everything I wanted and even more deliciously demanding than I thought. We were tortured in dance class, rigidly trained in the classics while also exploring the age of method acting. The only thing I missed at school was music. There were vocal training classes but no singing. I found some side jobs sitting in with house bands at places like the Purple Onion, where Jim Neighbors had gotten his start. I must have sung, "I left My Heart in San Francisco "a thousand times.

I had a sweet little studio apartment with a murphy bed that pulled down out of the wall, a short keyboard piano, and of course my little dog Kermit. Always the entrepreneur, I saw an opportunity in a small unused closet on the 4th floor of the conservatory. I asked if I could run a small lunch café out of it. With permission granted, I started "The 3 Penny Pantry." Nightly I baked homemade quiche (grandma's secret recipe) sandwiches and "Bieler's" soup – a special request of one of the directors. This gave me spending money. I hired Jim, a close friend from college to run the café. Jim had relocated to San Francisco following an immersion into a cult like worship group led by Sun Myung Moon of the Unification

Church. It was fun and I enjoyed writing music, acting, singing, and living life to the fullest. I was 21 years old and my life seemed perfect. At the end of our first year our class of 43 was cut down to 21. At year 3 those that remained were considered for a position with the professional theatre company.

I went home for the summer to await the final cut decisions. While I was home, I auditioned for and landed the leading role as Sally Bowles in Cabaret at an equity-waiver venue in North Hollywood called "The Agape Theatre." It was headed by Director Panos Christi and funded by Edna Glover, the wife of Myer Mishkin. I weighed the prospect of playing very small roles for years at the Geary Theatre against playing the role of a lifetime as Sally. Always an impatient woman, it wasn't hard to choose. The production was well received, and I ended up playing the role in several road companies over the next couple of years. I also won a Drama Logue Award for my portrayal of Jill in "Equus." Jill was a stable girl who unlocked the lust and childhood trauma of the leading man. It was a great role and I loved using an English accent for the second time. I was in the same award category as Joanne Worley that year for her excellent portrayal of the title role in "Mame." I was starstruck to get the nod for the award. Surely this would lead me to my big break!

I rented an upstairs apartment in Hollywood with some friends when I got the role in Cabaret.

As the play was equity waiver, I was not being paid, so I got a job on Sunset Boulevard waiting tables at a nice French restaurant. It was common for actors in Hollywood to perform without pay in local productions. Then they could invite producers and casting directors to see them perform and hopefully land a paying gig in TV or movies. My real love was for the stage and many advised me I really belonged in New York. But for some reason, I just did not feel called to the East Coast.

I was eating an ice cream cone while filling my car at a gas station on the corner of Sunset and Vine. A man pulled alongside me in a beautiful light tan Excalibur, Series IV. It literally sparkled. The gray haired distinguished looking man asked me, "Can I have a bite of your ice cream cone?" I instantly quipped back; "Can I have a bite of your car?" He thought that was funny.

We got to talking. He was much older than me. I was 23 years old and he was in his mid to late 40's. He asked me if I was a model (a common come on- line in the day) and I told him no, but that I was an actress. His name was Jerry (same as my dad) Schwartz. He asked me if he and his girlfriend could buy me dinner that night. I told him I was performing in a play but maybe drinks later?

Jerry's curiosity was apparent. He asked if they could come to see the play? I told him that of course they could. I felt rather relieved that he had a girlfriend and that they would be coming together. When I told him that it was "Cabaret" he shared that he knew Liza Minnelli very well and that she frequently came over to his house for parties and sang at the piano. That got my attention. Maybe this man could help my career!

Jerry and his girlfriend, Beth, came to the show that night as promised. She was a bright and intelligent woman, much younger than him but probably 10 years my senior. She shared that she was a paralegal. They both enjoyed the show and asked if they could take me out for a bite to eat. Of course, I agreed, and before long we were sitting at the famous hotspot, Chasens in West Hollywood. Chasens was a restaurant that long served the Hollywood elite in a structure along Doheny and Beverly. That is where Ronald Reagan proposed to his second wife, Nancy. Jimmy Stewart had booked the whole place for his bachelor party. Every star of the era went there. I never thought I would have ever set foot in the place. Many business deals were made in the red leather upholstered booths.

I noted one of my favorite actresses, Emmy Award winning Cloris Leachman in a corner booth. When I mentioned that to Jerry, he insisted on taking me over to her booth and introducing us. I had been so inspired by her in The Last Picture Show for which she won an Academy Award. Also, I had long admired her comedic abilities on the Mary Tyler Moore Show and as the terrifying housekeeper in Young Frankenstein.

I was in disbelief that this was all happening to me in one day. Cloris was very hospitable and scooched over in her booth to make room for us to squeeze in. When Jerry boasted that he had just seen me in Cabaret she told me a personal story about how she had been slated to audition for the film, "I am a Camera," the non-musical version of Cabaret and where the leading role had come from. Cloris said she had not felt like going to work that day and blew off the audition and the part went to the magnificent Julie Harris, who went on to be nominated for a Best Actress award for Best Foreign Film Actress (BAFTA). As she sipped her martini, she laughed and said, "Oh, honey, if only I had it all to do again!"

The following several months were a whirl wind to me. Jerry took me everywhere he thought a young actress should be seen and heard. I remember lounging atop a grand piano at Simply Blues, a jazz club up high on the skyline singing, "When Sunny Gets Blue" to Chaka Kahn, and rubbing elbows with Ella Fitzgerald at a nightclub in the valley where I sat in with bass player John Patitucci and newcomer, Dianne Reeves.

All the while I was performing in Cabaret. The late nights took a toll on my vocal cords. The play was demanding with my character singing 11 songs in the production along with carrying a good deal of the dialogue. I was almost always on stage. I needed to have hot tea with lemon and saltwater to gargle between scenes. There is a scene where Sally swallows a prairie oyster, a raw egg with Worcestershire sauce in it. This remedy was supposedly good for her frequent hangovers. Being that method acting was at my core, I never considered faking it. And the response from the crowd more than made up for the discomfort and taste. But it was hard to sing afterward with that coating on my throat, so we took to spiking the mixture a bit with cognac to cut through the phlegm.

Jerry was concerned and took me to see Liza Minnelli's throat doctor. I couldn't believe Jerry was taking such good care of me at his own expense. I was sure this doctor charged fees I could never afford! He diagnosed some nodes showing up on my vocal cords and treated me until I recovered, all on Jerry's bill. By this time, I had been to Jerry's luxurious house on several occasions and had noted there was an autographed picture of Liza on his piano, as he had promised. I had also been told by Jerry that he owned the rights to the play, "Oliver." He told me that he was grooming me to take over the leading role of Nancy in a running production in London.

All the while, Jerry never put a hand on me or acted in any way like he was interested in me romantically or physically. He flirted playfully, but that was all. I saw him very much as a father figure. On many occasions Beth would join us on our escapades, and everything really appeared to be on the up and up. My skeptical mother even took me shopping to purchase clothes for London – chic grown up clothes. Mom had a flair for classy. We got my passport in order and plans were being made for my first trip out of the country. Cabaret had ended its very successful run and I was ready for my first big break!

A week before I was to leave, Jerry invited me over for a farewell dinner at his house. Beth would be there as well, and we would toast to my future success. I knew this man a full 8 months by now and fully trusted him. I showed up at the appointed time and noticed right off that something seemed off between him and Beth. Our dinner seemed a bit strained and I could not figure out what was going on. I assumed maybe they had had a fight or disagreement and that they had not wanted to cancel because it was our last night together. And then it became apparent that there was more than food on the menu. Jerry said that he hoped that I would have a very successful career and that he was proud to be a part of it and so was Beth. Beth nodded but would not look me in the eye.

Jerry came over close to me and mentioned that while he had always been a gentleman with me, he had always secretly been attracted to me and so was

Beth. I looked back and forth between them. Jerry was clearly coming on to me. He said, "I've done a great deal for you this year and maybe you wouldn't mind doing something for me…?"

I felt like I had been punched in the stomach. I was so devastated. Someone I thought really believed in me for my talent told me that indeed there would be a condition. I was to have sex with them. I was shocked and offended. The whole thing had just been a set-up and a very deceptive plot. Jerry had been toying with me all along. I told them that I would never trade myself for any part and ran out of there in tears.

My trip was cancelled. I became an unemployed actress again.

There are other Hollywood stories that were indicative of the reality of the "Casting Couch" as we called it back then. Seemed like someone was always saying that they knew someone who could help your career and then there would be a business dinner that turned into a date with benefits. It was how the game was played. Young actresses were at the mercy of powerful men who could make or break their careers. But as I was soon to find out there were the good guys as well.

I had received another offer of employment when I was performing in Cabaret. A film producer hired me for my first independent film, titled "The Necklace" by Guy de Maupassant. I played Mathilde Loisel, a lower middle-class woman who had always believed it was an accident of fate that she was not in a high state of aristocracy. She borrows and loses a pearl necklace to wear to a party in order to impress. Rather than confess the loss of the necklace, she purchases a replacement of the necklace for the socialite who lent it to her and spends the next 2 decades scrubbing floors to pay it back. In the end she ultimately finds out that the original necklace was a fake, and that she paid a high price for her stubborn pride.

It was my first film and I was very nervous, having only taken a few film classes in college. The script was good and allowed me to explore everything from the desperation of poverty to the grandiosity of the elite. There was even a grand ballroom scene where I danced the night away with a handsome suitor. The scene had a Cinderella-esque like quality. The costumes were gorgeous, and I was fitted for them on the lot of Paramount Studios. The story was set in 1880 and so the costumes were elaborate and complicated.

On my first day on set, I dressed for the first scene. Mathilde was daydreaming unhappily about her station in life. The script called for me to be eating a box of bonbons, but the Director had fallen in love with my little dog, Kermit. Instead of eating bonbons, he inserted Kermit as a lap dog I stroked in the scene. Unfortunately, Kermit was all black and photographed like an inkblot, so it took quite a while to get the lighting correct. As we finally were ready to begin, the Director of Photography, Steven Dubin, peered out at me from behind the camera and said, "Excuse me, but are those period contact lenses?" I was horrified! Had I really been that stupid to forget a fact like that? Of course, there were no contacts in 1880! As I flustered, he broke out in a big grin and said, "I'm just messing with you. No one is going to notice!"

It was the beginning of a relationship that would last nearly four years. Steven was a charismatic, very talented man who had moved to LA from Baltimore, Maryland to pursue his dreams in the film industry. We subsequently worked on a couple of other small industrial films together. He worked all the time and had built up a tremendous resume that would include Director of Photography on "The Unsinkable Molly Brown." He was eight years older than me, tall with beautiful dark brown eyes and a groomed beard. I fell in love with his dry sense of humor, his business talent, and his musical abilities. He played guitar and piano and I would sing with him when his group of friends would gather for meals and fellowship. We never lived together in all the years of our relationship. Both of us lived separately in our own apartments by this time. He lived up in Laurel Canyon and I had a studio apartment in Silver Lake.

On the heels of this film, I was cast as Jill Mason in a play called, "Equus" by Peter Shaffer.

The play told the story of a psychiatrist who attempts to treat a young man who has a pathological religious fascination with horses. A passionate and obsessive horse lover, the young man, Alan, blinds 6 horses to the horror and surprise of his family. Jill is a stable hand and befriends the confused Alan, trying to lure him out of his shell. They share a scene together in the barn with the horses where Jill seduces him, and it is his extreme reaction to this partnering that leads him to attack the horses because of what they have seen. The play called for both actors to be naked in this scene. I accepted the role in part to challenge myself to get over my body image issues. I felt that if I could play this part and not be aware of being so exposed, it would be a test of my talent and ability to completely immerse myself in a role.

The play was performed "in the round," where the audience surrounds the stage, which gave implied space. It would be the doctor's office or the barn, and we used very few set pieces. The horses were played by supporting cast members who wore horse head pieces made of wire and walked on raised horse hooves. It was a beautiful production, and the lighting for our nude scene was very tastefully done in shadows. The play was well received. The young man who played the lead role and me, were nominated for Drama Logue Awards for Best Actor and Best Supporting Actress. A producer picked up the show and moved it to Long

Beach where we continued an extended run of the show in a larger theatre.

All this time, I was beating the pavement looking for an agent to represent me. I had my headshots, my experience, my local live performances, and even some film work but I could not get signed. It was very frustrating. I heard once again that I should consider moving to New York. But felt like at this point, it would be too hard to start over back east. My relationship with Steven was failing. I decided to throw in the towel and move to North Carolina where a good friend of mine lived. It was a drastic move, but I was ready to bring my acting career to an end.

The cast of Equus knew about my decision. When we had our final cast party, it was also somewhat of a farewell party for me. Yet, there was a well-known casting director at the party. This man had come to multiple performances of Equus. This casting director liked to hang out with us after the shows. His name was David Graham, and he worked for David Powers, an Emmy Award winning TV Director and Producer. Powers directed the Carol Burnett show for its entire 10-year run. When I met Graham, he was casting Three's Company. Near the end of the party he got up to leave and asked me to join him outside. As we said our goodbyes, he said to me, "Je'net, I don't want you to give up yet. I want you to promise me you will stick around for at least another couple of months. Can you do that for me?" Of course, I knew how powerful he was in the industry. Through some tears, I agreed to try and wait it out. He put out his hand as if to shake on a deal and said, "Look maybe this will help you make ends meet, but don't tell anyone about it, okay?"

After he left, I went into the restroom at the party and opened the small paper in my hand. It was a check for $2,000! That amount of money seemed like a fortune to me in 1983. It was certainly enough to pay rent and expenses for a few months. I was moved by his generosity. But even more, I was moved by the fact that this very important man believed in my talent to this extent. He wanted nothing in return.

In fact, he was the one who helped me move forward. He got me auditions for Happy Days, Mr. Belvedere, MASH and cast me in an episode of Three's Company. I made more money on that one episode of Three's Company than I had made in all my years of stage acting. I will always remember Dave Graham for what he did for my self-confidence and self-worth.

Chapter 8
Rebound Romance

Steven and I were struggling through an on-again off-again break up. Just when we thought we had separated for the last time something would bring us back together. We were "on a break" when I started to rehearse for the revival of "Equus" in Long Beach. Steven had missed the original production as he was sitting Shiva, a Jewish mourning ritual, with his family back in Maine. I was running lines one afternoon on the stage. When I looked up, I saw Steven standing in the back of the theatre. He said he felt bad that he never saw me in the show for which I had won an award for my performance. He went on to say he wanted to make up for it. I was so in love with him. That's all it took. We were on-again throughout the run of that show. I began to believe that we could overcome the religious divide. When Steven invited me on a road trip to Santa Barbara, I was sure that he was going to propose.

I remember the dress I wore, a sweet knee length white dress with red polka dots, a bright red belt and a playful neckline. The circle skirt was made of chiffon and blew around seductively as we walked hand in hand along the pier. He treated me to a beautiful champagne brunch. As usual, he was incredibly fun and easy to be with. He had an extraordinary gift for telling stories. I was on pins and needles waiting for the big moment. On our road trip home, it was clear that he had not planned an engagement. He just planned a special romantic afternoon. I was crushed.

I cried in the car on the way back, and Steven was perplexed. I came to the hard realization that this relationship would never move forward if it wasn't going to move forward now. After 4 years, we knew all we needed to know about each other to look at the future and take the next step. But if Steven wasn't there now, I knew he never would be. This time it was me who called it off. And I vowed to stay strong.

Steven had never actually made any kind of monogamous promise to me. I don't think that was so that he could play around, but to keep a wall up between us when it came to commitment. He never went out on me, and I had no reason to believe there was anyone else he was seeing while we were dating. The fact that he didn't want a promise from me to do the same just frustrated me. I would have gladly committed but that was not his thing. When I felt particularly insecure, I would go out with other men to try to get under his skin in the hope it might make him jealous.

There were three other men that regularly called me up for a date. And, more to prove a point, I occasionally accepted their offers. One of the men was a very wealthy doctor who drove a Maserati. He flew me to Maui with him for a summer vacation. Another close friend, Ken Kravitz, owned the first music studio I recorded at (Hit City West). He made his affection for me clear. He took me to so many nice restaurants and special events. We spent many late nights drinking cognac and playing scrabble.

And then there was Alan. I met Alan several times when I went to see my brother play music. Alan was a jazz drummer and incredibly talented. Alan was small, wiry and intense. He could brighten a room when he finally loosened up and smiled. He heard things between the beats and embellished with sounds that I hadn't heard come from a drum section before. I was mesmerized when he played. That said, he was also terribly shy. He asked for and received my phone number, but when he would call to ask me out, he would just freeze. I can remember these long painful silences between one-word answers to questions I would throw out at him. I tried my best to make conversation with him. He just could never make it happen and I never dated him. Yet, he consistently called me every month or so, never giving up. Impressive, I thought. He never gives up.

So, when Steven and I finally broke up for good, I relented and finally made my first date with Alan. He surprised me by offering to make me dinner at his place. He shared a house in North Hollywood with 3 other musicians. Alan was a vegan at that time. He cooked Millet Loaf, a vegetarian version of a meatloaf. I was skeptical about how this dinner would turn out, but it was darn good. I was surprised we had a lot to say to one another and had a lot in common. A much different kind of man than Steven, but he put his arm around me as we walked up the driveway to my place. He surprised me with a sudden confidence I didn't expect from him.

When Alan asked me to marry him 6 months later, I readily accepted. Unbeknownst to me, Steven was getting engaged to a woman who was a writer on a game show. Within a year of breaking up, we were both married….to someone else.

Chapter 9
Marriage & Motherhood

On a beautiful March afternoon, Alan and I were wed at the Orcutt Ranch in Rose Hills. We said our vows in the rose garden. I wore a simple long lacey gown with flowers in my hair. My stepdad, David, walked me down the aisle. My nephew, Jerome, was the ring bearer. My mom arranged the whole thing with a reception at a country club nearby. The crowd was largely made up of musicians, actors, and business friends of my mom and David. My brother was Alan's best man.

Alan and I planned for a hippy honeymoon. We were to stay at a bed and breakfast in Ojai and then drive up to Big Sur. We set off in his orange Volkswagen Bus. We were on such a cloud of happiness that neither of us noticed for several hours that we had headed south instead of north on the highway. Turning around and heading back set us back over 5 hours. It was dark when we entered Ojai. The bed and breakfast turned out to be disappointing. It turned out to be a small room with little privacy. We shared a bath down the hall.

I sat on the chenille bedspread and the tears just started to flow down my cheeks. This is not what I pictured for our wedding night.

After some deliberation, we made the decision to head up to Santa Barbara where we thought we would be able to find something a bit more acceptable for newlyweds. The Bed and Breakfast owners were very nice about it. They looked up some hotels in Santa Barbara and called to make our reservation ahead of time. When we finally arrived in Santa Barbara, we were tired, and Alan had a tension headache. He headed to the bath hoping to soothe the pain, and we both fell asleep without touching one another.

It was an ill-fated trip, perhaps a precursor to our marriage. The van broke down several miles north of Santa Barbara two days later. We ended up spending the next 5 days in a cheap motel in Morro Bay. The news on the van wasn't good and the repairs basically ate up our entire honeymoon budget. That said, you could break down in a worse town than Morro Bay. We made the best of it by spending as much time outside of our motel room as possible. We watched sea otters and went to the bird sanctuary. When the van was fixed, we drove into Solvang for the last two nights. We only had enough money to stay one night in a motel. The other night we spent in the back of the van happy as clams while feasting on a dinner of tequila and popcorn.

I had a job working with an art director, Roger Collins. He was famous for the "Bull in A China Shop" commercial. The job paid very well. When I became pregnant, they were more progressive than most employers in those days. They allowed me to bring little Jeremy to work with me and gave me a place to nurse him well before it was fashionable. Alan worked at the local Tower Records for minimum wage. We found a cute little house in Alta Dena and settled into being parents.

We found a neighborhood daycare when Jeremy was about 1 year old. At that same time, I took a new job at Wilhelmina Artists in Hollywood. I started in an entry level position but worked my way into a promotion before long. I was already preparing the weekly payroll for our talent each week. Then I received training to renegotiate contracts with returning artists like Sela Ward and Heather Locklear. I earned the title of Director of Business Affairs. Yet, I missed performing so much that it hurt.

I let my circles know I was looking for another gig. I did some community theater in Alta Dena and started to sing in the clubs again. I kept my eye on the Drama Logue for audition opportunities.

I also started my own side business, Sitting Pretty. I had started to pet sit for a few folks in my area, and really enjoyed the critters I got to hang with. This was the beginning of the era when people had begun to publicly treat their pets as family, and I had very little competition in my area. It was a great second income. Also, it gave me a nice opportunity to get a little time to myself or with a friend. I went on day trip getaways with my best friend, Linda Turner, while our boys, also best friends, hung out with their dads. Before long, my business was making a little bit of a local splash. The neighborhood paper ran a story about my business. The paper included a picture of me reading a book to a cock-a-too named, "Bobbity". That boosted business quite a bit and I found myself even having to turn work away. Pet owners loved me. They were constantly surprised that their pets, especially dogs, took to me so quickly. What they didn't know was that I had a secret. I (almost) never washed the pants I wore to meet new pets. So many animals had slobbered on those pants that they were irresistible! I came off as a pet-whisperer!

Before long I got a call from a theatre buddy. Director Panos Christi, who had directed me in Cabaret. He told me he was working on a new project and thought I should audition. The show was called, "Homeless, A Street Opera," and Panos thought I should try out for the part of Tess.

Chapter 10
Homeless, a Street Opera

I was so excited to be coming back to the stage with my favorite director and friend, Panos Christi. A full-blooded Greek, he was pensive, artistic, passionate and an insatiable flirt. He always seemed to teeter between moody and playful with a rare type of mischief that was contagious. As a director he had great insight into the characters of a play while still allowing his actors to find their own way into the soul of the lives they would temporarily inhabit.

I was cast in one of the leading roles, Tess, a streetwalker who was 8 months pregnant and addicted to heroin. Other cast members represented other homeless stereotypes; the bag lady, the flamboyant gay man, the pimp, the speed freak and the young runaway. The issue of homelessness was still a largely unreported dark story that was rarely talked about on the news. Skid row in Los Angeles was just beginning to grow into its name. More and more people were seen on park benches and sleeping on the concrete. It was becoming topical and we wanted to represent the stories of these folks with dignity.

Tess was the product of an abusive home, a victim of her own father who started to molest her at the age of four. Her mother had looked the other way and not protected her. Sound familiar? Keep in mind at this time I still had no surfaced memories of the abuse I had endured. Once again, I was cast in a role that had some connection to trauma I had endured as a child. The part hit an emotional nerve for me. One of songs I sang was about the actual act of incest and even with how wrong Tess knew it was, she still longed for the love of her father.

One of Tess's ballads still haunts me. How could I sing this and not connect to my earlier abuse?

"Daddy please come home, your little girl is so cold, and so alone, daddy please come home. Home is not a place, it's in the sight of daddy's face, the feel of your embrace, your breath upon my face...Home is in your arms, in your daddy's smile... beneath your pulsing hips..."

I literally sang that while on the stage floor, imitating my father laying on top of me. The show was quite graphic, but it was somewhat hip to shock this audience in that era. Method actors were bringing a stark reality to their roles, smoking real cigarettes on stage, unafraid of nudity and graphic sex scenes.

In this role I shot up heroin. With grim realism I gave birth with horrifying screams. I died a desperate death on stage while singing the whole thing. After all, it was a "light" opera. The show received extremely good reviews, but not too many of the general public wanted to come and see a show about the seedy lives of the homeless. We closed after only a few months.

My mother had come to see the show, as had my stepfather and my brother. There was quite a bit of swearing in the show. I had warned my mom about that. When she never really said too much to me about the play or my performance, I assumed it was because she thought the show itself was too obscene for comment. To be fair it was raw. So, I didn't think much of the lack of her usual post show commentary.

My brother was likewise quiet. It was months after the show closed that he asked me to meet him for breakfast. I had not seen him for quite a while. Now in our thirties we managed a guarded adult relationship.

When I walked in the restaurant that morning, I could tell that something was very wrong. Jack looked pale and upset, as if he had recently been crying. He opened his mouth and started talking and I felt the room pull away. I can't even remember exactly what he said, but I remember that he irrevocably opened a door to the past that would never be closed again. The play had blown the cover off Jack's locked memories. As he shared those memories with me, I retreated further and further away.

What I experienced in a matter of minutes was a lifetime of secrets all let out of a Pandora's box at once. So many things were going through my mind that I couldn't grab on to any of them. Jack talked about how we used to touch each other and ourselves in the back seat of the family car. Our parents were in the front seat. Were they aware? As children that behavior had unbelievably seemed natural and unremarkable to the both of us. What did that say about us and the childhood we had lived? There were other things and other memories he shared.

My life as I thought I knew it was changed forever. I left that restaurant a different person.

Chapter 11
Losing My Grip

I drove home in a fog. Tears were rolling down my cheeks, but I emotionally could not feel anything other than the sensation of being light-headed.

I tried to talk to my husband, Alan, about what Jack had shared with me. He was simply unprepared for anything this horrible. He had grown up in a very traditional family that had immigrated from Scotland. We shared the experience of having both lost our fathers early in life. That tragedy was the worst thing he had ever endured. He was compassionate but didn't know how to support me. His best advice was to try and put it behind me. To him, this was something that had happened a very long time ago. He couldn't really understand how it could be so devastating for me when it rose to the surface.

I pulled back from this relationship and other relationships. I received the same or similar advice from friends. Childhood incest was not a topic of conversation in any circle that I interacted with. I was in what I considered to be a pretty relevant and progressive crowd.

I called my mother a few days after Jack and I had talked. She did not answer the phone and so I left her a message. She did not immediately respond so I continued to leave several other voice messages over the next week. By this time, she and I had been in the habit of talking every few days and meeting for lunch 2 to 3 times per month. A lot of our past struggles had been put behind us. As the grandmother to my son, she and I found common ground. But the absence of a return phone call was ominous and ever present. Almost 6 months later, I got up the nerve to call her one more time. She finally talked to me.

I will never forget how that phone call affected me and how I felt when it was over. I hoped to hear that she was sorry about what had happened to me and for not seeing it or stopping it. I hung on to the idea that she was sifting through her own painful memories like me and was embarrassed to face me.

Instead, she finally said to me, "I've been meaning to call you Je'net, but I didn't know what to say. I just can't believe that I could marry a man who could do such a thing."

This sentence turned in toward herself and made no room for me. She thought how it was so hard for her to believe or cope with the idea that she could have been such a fool to marry my dad. She felt how difficult it was for her to come to terms with it. In fact, her feelings were a mirror of what I had faced all my life. Could she really be more obsessed with how this affected HER? Could she have no sympathy or compassion for what I, a defenseless child had gone through? She had refused to see it then and refused the see it now as well.

There was no, "I'm so sorry this happened to you honey" or "I'm so sorry" or "I can't believe I didn't see this," and certainly not a "Baby, how can I help support you?"

It felt more like she didn't believe me and that the abuse surely never really happened. She didn't want to talk about it. She didn't want anyone to know. Like everyone else, she seemed to want the past to stay in the past.

With the truth right in front of her, and even backed up by her favorite child, my brother, she abandoned her daughter once again.

Because she had subsequently married a man that had worked with my father, and still socialized with many of the same people that she had while married to him, she was desperately afraid that this story would get out. She asked me if I had shared this with anyone, and did I plan to? The whole conversation was about how to keep this a secret.

I quietly hung up the phone without answering any of her questions.

Not brave enough to view them, I had a box of 8-millimeter films from my childhood, home movies of the family together. But now I pulled the dusty box from the back of my closet and started to watch them one after the other. I saw a little girl who was anxious and precocious, that was clearly close to tears in many of these films without there really being a reason for it. In some I was captured sobbing, but no one comforted me. I saw my mom, often with a quizzical look on her face and a brother who seemed disconnected and distant. My father was the one holding the camera. There was no footage where he was in frame with his family. Like a documentary without truth or answers, I watched and drifted away again.

I started to spiral. I turned to my old friend, cocaine. The drug became my only place of no pain. It seemed the only way to get through the day and make it manageable. The depth of what had happened to me seemed be like an enormous boulder that sat on my chest, the kind of weight that was my father on top of me. As the memories surfaced, each one more unbearable than the last, the ONLY thing that took it away was to keep putting cocaine up my nose. It kept me at a safe distance away from the ache that seemed to emanate from my very soul. In the weeks and months to come, I became what is known as a functional addict. I held down a job, a marriage, and the parenting of a young son by pushing through the day. But the moment that he was down for the night or that I had a few empty hours when I might think (which would lead me to feel) I medicated. When this finally caught up with me, I fell into the sordid life of a drug addict. Nothing was off the table in order to get high and escape my pain.

I used cocaine almost daily to get me up and behaving like an involved and present mom. I used it to get me through the long workdays. I used it on the weekends to turn them into escapes. I took lots of new pet sitting jobs so that I could isolate and use. Sometimes I would rent a motel room for a night and say I was pet sitting. I didn't think that my use was apparent to anyone most of the time, but I knew that the drug was serving a whole new purpose for me. I began to hang out with people that used it a lot themselves to normalize my own behavior.

I remember one night in a motel in Van Nuys. I had gone through my mind-numbing stash and medicated what I had done to get it. It involved paying for my drugs with some dollar bills wrapped around Monopoly money. The drug dealer had chased me up the street yelling at me that he would cut my throat if he ever saw me again.

Suddenly aware that I could die using this drug, I looked up an 800 number to Cocaine Anonymous. I made the phone call and was assured that someone was on their way to my motel to rescue me and take me to a meeting. Instead, a man from the hotline showed up with rock cocaine. He got high with me and raped me. Then he tossed the remainder of the stash on the shag carpet saying, "There you go bitch! Do the dog, you hopeless piece of shit." He knew that an addict would search on their hands and knees for the pieces of crack and smoke whatever they came across in the process.

Before long, I lost my job as Director of Business Affairs with Wilhelmina Artists. I often worked late hours by myself in the high-rise building in Hollywood. I used to be careful about using the restroom to pull out my vile of cocaine but got sloppy about it as time went on.

My boss, Phillip, and I were in the same group counseling sessions on a weekly basis. That's how we had met. I know that my sharing in this group had become a lot to handle. One day he pulled me in his office and said he was letting me go. He was nice about it. He didn't call me out on anything specific and he truly looked sad as he delivered the news.

But I knew I was losing my grip.

I recently watched a movie called, "Beautiful Boy." The movie is about a young man who fell into a life of addiction. His parents tried everything as soon as they realized what was going on in order to save him. I was shaken and in tears remembering my own journey. I left the theatre grasping my husband's hand tightly in an effort to hold it together in front of our daughter.

The truth was that from 3 years old *no one* had ever tried to save me. No one rescued me from the abuse I suffered as a child. No one helped me get the therapy I needed to deal with my resurfacing memories. My mom had shut it down once in high school, so I knew she wouldn't help me now. I found my own therapist in North Hollywood. I couldn't begin to pay the center for the cost of the number of sessions I needed. Once they understood what I was trying to cope with, the center took me on at no charge. Incredibly, my mom and brother tried to disrupt my therapy. They called the center and told my counselor that I was just a drug addict and not worthy or ready to accept her help. I was there, wasn't I?

I remember my therapist calling me to tell me this. She said, "I'm so sorry Je'net. I have to tell you something that just happened, but I want you to know first, I am not going to stop helping you. I promise!" Then she laid out what my family members had said. I was devastated. Did they need to keep the secrets buried so badly that they would actively try to stop me from getting help? While I continued to go to my sessions there seemed to be no point.

As I watched this movie about how many times the father, played by Steve Carell, tried to help his son, it just seemed to settle in deeper for me how my family never once tried to offer me a drug rehab or support me to stop using. My family never offered me any kind of emotional support. They just judged me seeing only the drugs. They wanted the drugs to be the problem and not the horrible abuse I had suffered. They were single mindedly focused on one thing. They wanted to silence me and keep this awful secret! My own family wanted to put a wall between me and the difficult journey of healing.

To be fair, they did ONCE offer me a quick fix from a hypnotherapist. This "professional" met with me for an hour. Then he told me that he only needed one 6-hour session to pull up all my unsurfaced memories and get me past them. In an off-handed manner, he told me that he would meet with me after hours at his office.

The Doctor explained, "You're likely to make a significant amount of noise. Most of my patients cry and even scream as I pull these memories up and out of them."

Casually, he went on to say that he didn't want any of the other office employees to call for the police. I was appalled and frightened. I wanted to remember but not this way. I declined this heartless attempt at making me face my past and "get over it." It seemed to be what everyone wanted. Again, I heard loud and clear, "It happened a long time ago" and "Why couldn't I just move on?"

Traumatized and terrified, I dragged myself into a motel room after a man had beaten me and left me with a horrible black eye. I called my brother, Jack. In desperation I begged him for help and for him to come and get me.

Jack, through *his* tears cried, "I'd like to help you but I… just…can't!" He quietly hung up on me.

I remember thinking, "When have you ever?"

I hit my head against the wall over and over trying to make my physical pain surpass the heartache and hopelessness I felt inside.

In the movie, Beautiful Boy, based on the book "Tweaked," the dad says this same thing to his son. The dad says, "I wish I could help you, but I just can't." But the dad in the movie said that *only* after he had supported several inpatient care programs and *many* attempts at rescuing his son. He labored over the loss of his beautiful boy.

It's just that no one ever did that for me. Everyone stood back. For them it was like watching a car accident in slow motion. I had been on my own fighting for survival since I could remember. With that desperate and fierce sense of survival, I eventually rose above it with the love of a kind-hearted person. I met him in a park, a stranger who thought I was worth the effort.

Chapter 12
The Rise

On January 24th, 1991, my friend Robin and I went to Anaheim for the NAMM show. NAMM stands for National Association of Musician Merchants. Well over 100,000 merchants, vendors and musicians attend each year to see the newest lines of musical instruments, equipment and services from all over the world. It is also quite a party attended by famous musicians like Peter Frampton, Gregg Allman, David Bowie, the Steve Miller Band, B.B. King, and Vince Gill, just to name a few. These talented personalities could often be seen candidly sitting in a booth playing a new guitar for fun and even composing on the spot. The atmosphere is energized with talent and dreams.

As part of the music industry, Robin worked as a Piano dealer. She attended the show with her sister from North Carolina and I was along for the ride. At the end of the first day we decided to get a cocktail at The Jolly Roger Hotel. Sitting on a stool in the lounge, I caught the eye of a tall handsome stranger at the far end of the room. At first glance, I thought it was Ted Nugent. He smiled at me as if asking for an invitation, and I did not disappoint. I nodded at the empty stool beside me and he made his way through the celebratory crowd.

He introduced himself to me. He wasn't Ted Nugent, but I thought he was just as good looking. He was tall and slim but muscular. Towering 7 inches over me at 5'11"and 180 pounds, he had long hair flying free down to the middle of his back. He was strikingly attractive. His eyes and smile, the best things about him, were bright and engaging. You almost couldn't help but like him on sight. In order to protect his anonymity and my safety, I won't share his name, but let's call him Grayson.

Grayson was marketing a product at the NAMM show that he had invented and patented. The product was made in Utah where Grayson lived. He assembled his product himself, literally in his living room, and shipped it all over the world. The way he talked he was closely connected to many A List stars in the music industry and on the brink of becoming a multi-millionaire.

Within the first 20 minutes of meeting me, and with a second cocktail on board, I was sharing stories with this guy and returning his flirtatious affection. We hit it off so well that 3 hours later we were sharing a bed.

As we began to become intimate, Grayson noticed a change in my demeanor. I had not been having relations with my husband, Alan, for over 6 months. I wanted to warn Grayson that I wasn't sure how I would respond to my first sexual encounter since my trauma had surfaced. When he felt me tense up, Grayson stopped touching me immediately and gave me space. I couldn't believe I was telling this stranger my story. I had just met him! Surely, he would find the door and just leave.

Remarkably, my story didn't faze him a bit. He was sensitive, understanding, and never once tried to minimize it or play down its significance. He shared that he knew several women who had gone through similar experiences and that I should feel comfortable talking to him about it. I relaxed and trusted him immediately.

I look back at it now and think, "Wow, he really had my number."

It was the best sex I had ever had up to this point in my life. Fun, intimate, a little dangerous and very gratifying. He was strong and physically took a commanding lead, while still managing to be gentle and generous. For the time I was with him, the rest of the world just fell away.

Intimacy with Grayson was natural and organic. We couldn't get enough of one another. We spent a good part of the next 3 days together before he had to return to his home state of Utah. He even managed to sneak me into the show, not an easy feat with the tight security at NAMM.

Over the next several months, Grayson and I would talk almost daily. Always a fan of the written page, I wrote him lengthy letters. Pages and pages of letters, pouring out my heart and my history. I would beg him to write back to me, but he would always sidestep the request. He said he had terrible handwriting and talking to me was so much better. When I did receive a letter from him it shocked me to see the extent of his poor spelling and grammar, almost like a 3rd grader. I joked with him about it and he said he had a reading disability and had never really written well. I felt horrible for bringing it up.

He laughed, "I told you I couldn't write!" But I could tell I hit a sore spot and should drop it. He explained, "I can think, and that's all that matters."

I was dying to see him in person again. He said that he wanted to come out to see me too but that finances were tight. He lived a humble life in Utah and never seemed to have the money for airfare. I didn't think twice about paying for his flight. I would sacrifice just about anything to see him. Travel to and from Utah wasn't very expensive and I put aside some of the cash I got from pet sitting to pay for him. Grayson promised that he would repay me as soon as some income came in from his product sales and I believed him.

He would fly out from Utah to stay with me when I had a pet sitting job for more than 3 days. I would plan an elaborate romantic escapade and we would drink champagne and play. We would connect with his friends in Orange County, people who raced motorcycles and played in bands. Grayson himself was a biker, and he would borrow a bike and take me on long rides to the beach and up the coast. He also played the drums quite well but, unlike Alan, he was into heavy metal and rock and roll.

Grayson could literally talk for hours at a time about subjects and controversial topics that none of my friends talked about. He theorized about the Vietnam war and about the real government involvement. He believed it was a diabolical plan to reduce the population of young men in the US, especially young men from disadvantaged backgrounds. He would share his theories with such authority and confidence, it was hard to contest, even though much of it sounded far-fetched.

He told me on many occasions that the police in Utah were specifically after him because of his unconventional behavior. He reported that they parked near his home and set up surveillance that included high powered hearing devices that could pick up conversations from blocks away. Frankly, this was a common paranoid theme for him. From his perspective, people always tried to take advantage of him and steal his ideas. Grayson shared numerous stories about how he had almost made it, but then was taken out by some villainous character who acted out of greed and jealousy. They robbed him of his deserved success. He proudly declared that he was on the top ten watch list with the local authorities who didn't appreciate his outspoken nature in a conservative Mormon community. He believed that people admired him for his high IQ and innovative thinking but were threatened by him. Grayson didn't like it when you challenged his theories. I learned not to challenge him. But that was okay. He was certainly entertaining, and I was charmed and fascinated with him.

I was so enchanted by him and already falling in love with him. Also, I felt so relieved that this man didn't see me as damaged goods. In fact, he complimented me often and generously. He said he had never met anyone like me, and that none of his old girlfriends could hold a candle to me.

"You have to come to Utah, so I can show you off," he would say.

It would always be a tearful goodbye at the airport. And it wasn't just me. He looked truly depressed and sad to leave when the time came. We were that annoying couple who couldn't stop kissing and groping each other at the gate.

Alan and I broke up officially. We were arguing one day, and it became physical. He pushed me away from him and as a result I lost my balance and fell backward. I hit my head and bruised my arm. He didn't mean to hurt me, but it was the straw that finally broke our failing marriage. I kicked him out of the house.

Our son, Jeremy, was confused and scared about the changes in our household. He had not seen Alan and I be affectionate with one another for quite a while. We both loved him tremendously and showed it all the time. Jeremy started to act up. He cried more than usual over a scraped knee or spilled cup of juice. Jeremy had a fear of spiders and became almost hysterical when he saw a bug that might fit the classification. I shared Jeremy's fear with Grayson. Grayson said the next time he was in town he would try and help Jeremy deal with his fear.

I arranged for Grayson to meet Jeremy. We staged it so we would just run into one another at the mall. I introduced Jeremy to my new friend, and we got some McDonalds together. I thought we carried it off as platonic friends, but it wasn't hard to notice the chemistry between the two of us and children are very perceptive. At one point, Grayson touched my hand. I brushed him away, but not quickly enough.

Jeremy started to misbehave, unusual for him in a public place. When he just wouldn't settle down, we left and got in our car to head home. On the way home he kept kicking the back of my seat. He started to throw things at me that were within his reach. I finally had to pull over and settle him down. His tantrum was full blown. Not at all the norm for this kid who usually displayed an easy-going personality. It took a good 20 minutes until he wore himself out and went to sleep.

So much for a good first impression.

Grayson and I decided that the truth was the best way forward. I told Alan that I had met someone new and that I did not see us getting back together. By this time Grayson and I were talking about living together. Would he move out to California? Or would I consider going to Utah?

Alan and I had "the talk" with Jeremy and it went about the way you would expect. Jeremy was 4 years old and couldn't understand the complexity of what we were saying. We just kept assuring him that even if daddy and mommy didn't live together, we would still be a family and we would always love him.

Grayson continued to visit every other month or so. He would come out to the house in Alta Dena and fix my car or mow the lawn, the Man stuff. He would try and engage Jeremy in those things. Grayson offered to show Jeremy how to be a big boy and fix mommy's car so he could do it for me when he was older. Jeremy warmed up a bit but was still standoffish. Grayson was the opposite of Alan in so many ways. He was loud when Alan had been soft spoken. He was handy with fixing things and liked physical challenges. Alan liked to read and listen to jazz.

One day I was in the kitchen fixing lunch when I heard a ruckus from the back yard. Jeremy was crying and yelling for me. Grayson was standing next to him focused on something on the ground. It was a spider. Jeremy was terrified and wanted Grayson to kill the spider. Grayson told Jeremy he needed to be the one to face his fears and deal with it.

He had given Jeremy his shoe and was pointing to the spider saying, "YOU have to kill the spider, Jeremy! Be a man! What if you had to protect your mom from the spider and I was not here? Go on…!"

Jeremy was getting hysterical. Brushing his tears away, he made a half-hearted swipe at the spider and it scurried towards him. I noticed then it was a black widow. He screamed and ran away. I screamed too and ran to swoop Jeremy up and away from the danger. I comforted him and soothed his little self. I glared at Grayson. I took Jeremy in the house to settle him down. Jeremy ate his lunch while watching cartoons. Before long he was immersed in his favorite show, Teenage Mutant Ninja Turtles.

Grayson laughed it off and told Jeremy, "Well, at least you tried kid!"

I was angry with him, but not for long. He instantly became softer and ingratiating. He shared that he was just trying to step in and give Jeremy some male role modeling.

"You gotta toughen him up Je'net. You don't want him to grow up soft."

Chapter 13
The Fall

It was the summer of 1992. Jeremy was to start kindergarten that fall. Grayson and I were still seeing each other whenever we could. More and more, Grayson would ask me for small amounts of money to help him pay off his manufacturers and buy the materials he needed to make and sell more of his product. He wouldn't come right out and ask me. He would just mention how much he wanted to see me but that every penny he made as a mechanic he was sinking into his business. He would incentivize me to offer him support.

Grayson was sly!

"If I could only get this order out and get paid, I could come see you and treat you to some nice dinners. Maybe get you a piece of jewelry or fly you here. But I don't have enough to cover the new die mold we need to start production."

I found myself offering to send him the money so that he could get his business back on track. But then there would be another expense and another. He was always behind and broke.

One night, Grayson called me. He was very excited! He and an affluent friend of his, Joe, had an opportunity to do something he had always dreamed of. They planned to open a nightclub in Salt Lake City. Grayson knew that he could make this a success with all his contacts in the music industry and with Joe's business sense. The two had apparently made a deal to renovate an old building downtown and turn it into a club. The plan was for Joe to buy the entire block of businesses complete with current tenants who would pay enough rent to cover the cost of the monthly mortgage. Their plan made the venue rent free. Joe had told Grayson that he could live in the building which used to be a large 3 story department store. They would use the 2 top floors for living quarters and office space. Then gut the downstairs to make room for the club.

Grayson was beside himself about this project. It would be the climax of his career and the best venture ever. Joe needed his connections in the music industry to make it happen. Grayson needed his money and so they would be partners.

He said, "Now we can be together Je'net. You have to move here and help me. You can even be a silent partner. Sell your pet sitting business and use it to move here and help me open this club!"

His excitement was infectious. I completely bought in sight unseen. This was the time for the move if we were going to get Jeremy set up in kindergarten in Utah before the school year started. Before long I had a buyer for Sitting Pretty, and I turned over that money to Grayson. I fully trusted that I would be a partner and investor in the club.

My husband, Alan, could not really put up a fight. He was struggling to stay afloat and was back living with his mom. He had taken a contract with a cruise line to play jazz and save some money. He would be gone off and on for 9 months. He couldn't fight for Jeremy under those circumstances.

My family thought it was a bad idea and so did most of my friends. But I didn't have a lot of time for friends anymore. Grayson didn't like that. Grayson would remind me how badly they had treated me and remind me that they didn't really care about me. I couldn't argue with any of that. I felt that my family would be relieved if I left California and moved away. They did nothing to persuade me differently.

Grayson started to want to know where I was and with whom. He would ask casually as if just interested in my day. He would tell me that he would call me at a certain time but leave me waiting for the call for hours. He would then check in from a party somewhere just to make sure I was at home. He told me that he would call me later. That was usually hours after I fell asleep. I often wondered if he was being faithful but comforted myself with the knowledge that I would be there in Utah with him soon. Then I would be on his arm at these parties fending off unwanted advances from other women.

From here the story becomes predictable. I never saw my money again. I never got any paperwork stating that I was an investor. I became isolated in Utah with only the friends that Grayson wanted me to have. When the money ran out, he insisted that I get a full-time job to pay my share of expenses. He would expect me to stay up all hours in order to assemble and package his product. It became clear that my opinions and contributions (other than financial) were unwelcome.

More and more evenings he would leave and not come home until daybreak. When he did, he was often drunk and high. Or manic, up all night fixing one of the many broken motorcycles in the garage. When he wanted me to be compliant, he would make drugs available to me, or let me know where to get them. He showed me how to smoke cocaine, and that became a monster that plagued me for the next several years. I became controlled by this drug and desperate for the escape it offered me in my misery. Crack cocaine will kill your soul.

One evening, I became especially angry at him for not coming home or calling me. I had made a special dinner for him for his birthday and it sat on the kitchen table for hours. When he finally came home, I tried to get him to make love to me, but he said he would need to shower first. That let me know he had been with someone else. I was sobbing and beating my fists at him. He dragged me out into the snow bare naked by the throat. He tossed me into a snow drift, went back into the house and locked the back door. I could hear him in the hot shower. I nearly froze before he let me back in.

Later, he would tell me that it had been my fault, that I knew he would be out working, and it wasn't any of my business where he was or who he was with.

Of course, there would be days when he was back to the old Grayson that I fell in love with. That's how he kept me hopeful that things would change. He would give me just enough attention and affection to get me smiling again. He would include me at a party with friends, take me and Jeremy out for a meal, or to a picnic at the park. But he controlled the money now, and I had nothing if he didn't give it to me. My paychecks were signed over to him and the welfare food stamps were turned over to him. This money seemed to always disappear, and he would bring home snacks he dug out of a dumpster for Jeremy and me.

The nightclub venture fell away. Most of the time he and his partner Joe were turning the rent money into drugs. They had parties with friends that sometimes lasted two or three days. Grayson would cold heartedly parade old and new girlfriends in front of me, most of whom were clearly as infatuated with him as I was. Why couldn't I just leave and go home?

I went to Utah with self-confidence and in love with a man I thought I would spend the rest of my life with. I went to Utah with him because my past abuse had not scared him off. In fact, Utah is one of the most notorious states for child abuse, and almost everyone I met there had a past that included incest or some other physical or psychological abuse.

Within 18 months I did not recognize the person I had become.

Chapter 14
Lay Down and Die

In June of 1993, I sent Jeremy home to spend the entire summer with Alan's mother, Grandma Margaret. I had finally designed a plan to leave Grayson and go back home. I needed a car for the trip and a longtime friend of mine, Avi, sent me $400 to buy an old Honda. The car needed a new clutch and some brakes. Grayson, who was "happy to see me go," agreed to prepare the car for the 558-mile journey.

I had been looking up want ads on the computer for employment in my field and found an opportunity in talent payment at an advertising company. I landed a phone screening with them and they promised me a second interview if I could come to California. They were hiring and said I sounded like a good fit. I was nervous about driving all that way on my own, but the old Je'net made a command appearance. I packed the car with what it would hold and left Grayson in the rearview mirror.

I got to Las Vegas that evening. The car had done well, and I was glad to put the Utah landscape behind me and pull into the city. I parked the car at a convenience store to use the bathroom and get a coffee. I had planned to drive all night, and this was to be my only rest stop for a quick meal.

I came back to the car, settled back behind the steering wheel, and turned the key in the ignition. I put the car in reverse and lifted off the brake, while putting my foot on the gas. Nothing happened! The engine just revved, and the gears wouldn't shift at all. I tried everything and was clearly in distress when some passerby stopped to pay attention.

One of them said, "Sounds like your clutch went out, honey."

I couldn't believe it. I did not have a contingency plan. I had bags of chips in my car, a big gulp and about $80.00. Just enough to drive straight through to LA. There was only one thing to do. I called Grayson from the phone in the convenience store.

He answered on the first ring. "Hey! How's it going? You make it to Vegas?"

I started crying, "Grayson, the car died! The clutch is out. I can't get it to run! I don't know what I'm going to do!"

He replied, "Yeah, that car's a piece of shit. I was surprised I could get it up and running at all. That's tough…."

"Can you come fix it? Please? You have to come get me! I don't have any money to fix this!"

There was a long pause on the other end.

"I just got rid of you Je'net. Why would I come help you? You could have stayed. This is on you."

And with that, he hung up.

I called back over and over for the next hour, but he never picked up again. I went out and sat in the car and locked the doors.

The owner of the convenience store came out to see why I was still in one of his few parking spaces. He said to me, "You can't just stay here, you know. You'll have to get this towed off my property."

By a miracle my AAA card was still valid. I called for a tow and within 25 minutes my car and all my belongings were towed to a repair shop. It was now 9pm and the shop was closed. This was as far as the tow truck driver could take me. He left me at the garage with my car.

I looked around. This didn't look like the Vegas I knew. There were no large hotels or casinos around, just seedy rooms for rent with a slot machine in the lobby. I took my small suitcase from the car and spent $21 for a room for the night. I ate a bag of Cheetos for dinner. I turned out the lights and just lay there. I could hear whoops of laughter, muffled sex, and the sounds of arguing men and women.

The next day I started calling everyone I had a phone number for. I kept track of the 25 cents per minute rate at the motel. I called my mom and brother to no avail. They still thought of me as a useless drug addict and didn't believe that I was literally in the situation that I said I was in. Grayson had made me call them for money repeatedly while I was living with him in Utah and they were no longer willing to help me. I then called my Aunt Donna who is my dad's sister, and she seemed to be willing to hear me out. She said she would see what she could do and call me back.

I didn't hear back from her. But I did get a call back from my brother, Jack. He screamed at me over the phone that I should be ashamed of myself for asking the family for help. He informed me that he was going to call everyone he and I knew and tell them not to help me either.

He said, "You need to hit bottom Je'net." And with that he hung up on me, again.

Hit bottom? Had I not?

I walked over to the garage for an update. The mechanic told me the car was in bad shape. In addition to the clutch, the car needed some other work before it would be street worthy, especially if I intended to drive it across the desert from Las Vegas to LA. The cost to repair the Honda was $825.00, an amount more than I could ever hope to pay.

The next three months were the darkest days of my entire life. There are few opportunities for a woman in her mid-thirties to make a buck in Vegas. Especially if you don't have the right clothes for an interview, a resume, or a place to clean up for a respectable job.

There are other ways to survive.... I had played roles that depicted those very professions. I stepped out of myself and into a role my mother had accused me of when I was 16. My whole life I had been told with words and actions that my best contribution to this world was on my back.

So, I laid down.

Chapter 15
Taking the Long Way Home

Ten weeks later I walked the 3 miles back to the garage where my car was held ransom. I had managed to save enough to finally get the car fixed but I wore the exhaustion on my face.

I was tired and had lost about 15 pounds. I had just what I could carry with me; a few changes of clothes, a single pair of jeans and two t-shirts. Also, I had a leather jacket and night clubbing attire that I needed to get into the casinos. By this time, I had been banned from Caesar's Palace and the MGM. Security was nice about it, but they didn't want me in their nicer bars. They had looked the other way when I had first arrived because I looked fresh and healthy. But later, it was clear that the life I was leading was hard on me. I no longer was able to class myself up enough to have them look the other way.

To my horror the garage took my money and then handed me another $240 bill for storage. They told me I had to pay that to get the car out of impound. I dropped into a chair in the dingy waiting room and put my face in my hands. I was ready to tell them to just keep the car, but all my and Jeremy's belongings were still in the back seat and trunk. I swallowed whatever pride I had left and called my Aunt Donna again.

I told her that I was still stuck in Vegas, but that I had gotten a job and was able to pay for the repairs. I left the part out about what kind of job it was. I just told her I worked in the casinos, which was true enough. I shared that I had to get out of Vegas and back to Utah in time to get Jeremy back in school two weeks later. This time she took pity on me and sent a money order for $400 through Western Union. I will always remain indebted to her for this. Years later I would send her the $400 with a grateful heart.

So, I headed back to Grayson with my tail tucked between my legs. I didn't tell him I was coming because I felt afraid that he would tell me not to return. I found another traveler. He was a 20 something young man named Ricky who was headed to Utah. He was willing to share gas money and we headed back to Salt Lake City together.

There are large stretches of highway between Las Vegas and Utah with no businesses, rest stops or diners. You could drive for an hour and only see a handful of other vehicles and nothing else. So, when my traveling buddy and I saw red lights in the rearview mirror, we couldn't imagine why we were being pulled over.

The officer came up slowly on the driver's side, scrutinizing the overloaded car, my passenger and me.

He said as he narrowed his eyes at Ricky, "Ma'am, I notice your tags are expired. May I please see your license and registration?"

"Oh God, no," I thought. I started to rummage through the glove box. I was going to register the car in LA when I got there but clearly that had not happened. I started to explain this to the officer, but he asked me if that were the case, why was I headed in the opposite direction? I didn't know how much to share about that and stuttered.

By now his partner was at the passenger window. He asked, "Do you have any drugs or weapons in the vehicle ma'am?"

Incredulously, I said, "What? Of course not, officer."

"Step out of the vehicle, Ma'am, and keep your hands where I can see them."

I did as I was told, as did Ricky, who was looking extremely nervous. The officers started poking around in the front seat.

I whispered to Ricky in a panic, "You don't have anything, do you?" He looked the other way and would not meet my gaze.

Within 5 minutes the officer pulled his head out from beneath the front passenger side seat. He held a small baggie with white powder in it.

He said as he eyeballed the two of us, "So what's this?"

I started to swear at Ricky, but he flipped it back on me and said it was mine. The officers then started to go through the car box by box. This took over an hour as we sat there in the hot sun. They opened every container, bag and box. They rummaged through all my things and left them in a heap at the side of the road. In the end, they didn't find any more drugs or weapons, but they had found an old pot pipe of mine deep in one of the duct taped boxes.

Ricky and I were both arrested for possession of drugs and paraphernalia.

They took us to a square bland looking holding facility out in the middle of nowhere. We were both fingerprinted there and put into separate cells. I never saw Ricky again. I was taken to the women's side of the jail. There were only four cells and I was the only female.

I surrendered to the situation and went to sleep. I didn't have any tears to shed. I was just defeated.

I couldn't believe this was happening to me, but on the other hand, wasn't it what I had come to expect?

I spent two weeks there before I was released. I was surprised at how clean it was and how good the food tasted. And there was so much of it! I think because everyone else at the jail was male, including the staff, the portions were enormous. It was a step up from where I had been staying in Vegas. The guards treated me with respect. I gained some weight and got an enormous amount of sleep. I felt relieved that every day did not start with survival mode. I did not worry about where I would spend the next night.

Eventually, I was told that Ricky had fessed up to his ownership of the drugs. He had admitted I was unaware he had anything on him when I offered him the shared ride. Ever my rescuer and unconditional friend, Avi paid my ticket for paraphernalia so that I could be released.

Rested and less haggard than two weeks before, I resumed my journey to Salt Lake City on my own.

Chapter 16
Life Imitating Art

I knew what I had to do. I had to return to Grayson and apologize to him for the way I had acted. Then play up to his ego and beg to be allowed to return. I needed to do this quickly as Jeremy was scheduled on a flight back to Utah in less than a week.

I played my part. The crazy thing was when I saw Grayson, I was at once mesmerized by him again. I was still in love with this man, but I could not for the life of me understand it. It made no sense. I had never allowed a man to dictate what I could and could not do or control me like this. I had absolutely no concept that I was in a classic domestic violence relationship. I groveled and took my lumps from him about how stupid I was to try and leave in the first place. I believed that it was all my doing. I fell right back into the rhythm of isolation and fear. I accepted that it was my fault things had gone wrong and my responsibility to make myself into someone that Grayson could love.

While I had been in Vegas the business dealings for the nightclub had gone sour with Joe. The tenants had been late or delinquent with their rent. Grayson accused Joe of keeping the money and not paying the mortgage. The two partners were on the outs with one another. Grayson had been evicted from the club and from what we had come to call our home.

As a result, Grayson had moved to a tiny house near the club over the summer. The dilapidated property had been condemned, but Grayson had managed to arrange a deal with the owner to fix it up in return for free rent. He put up a wall in the living room to section off a space for Jeremy to sleep. The space was diminutive so Grayson built a bunk bed with a ladder to the top for sleeping. This gave Jeremy a small play area underneath. Then I hung a curtain over the open-door frame.

The shack had a decided lean to it. In fact, if you put a glass on the floor in the kitchen it would roll from one end to the other. The foundation itself really needed to be repaired, but the house would have to be leveled. Leveling a house was beyond Grayson's construction abilities. Other than the living room there was a kitchen, one bedroom and a tiny bathroom.

It was very different from the club where the generous office space we used for bedrooms had more than 350 square feet. The bathrooms on each floor were built for the use of 15 to 20 employees at a time, but there were no showers. We used to take showers on the rooftop behind some shower curtains with a garden sprinkler head screwed on a hose connected to the hot water from the 3rd floor bathroom. While the bathroom in the lopsided shack was so small you could barely turn around, the indoor shower was a plus, especially in the winter.

Grayson showed some grace and we mended our fences enough to make life bearable. It was one of the seasons when I thought there might be a chance to make things better, like they used to be when we first met in California. We headed into the holiday season in better spirits. I stopped complaining about his late nights and made sure I was around for his calls. I had a job selling family films through a telemarketing company. I handed my paychecks to Grayson like before. I accepted his put downs and criticisms and learned to steer clear when he got manic.

January found us planning to return to the NAMM show together. Jeremy would go with us and see his dad for a few days as he had not seen him over Christmas yet. Grayson was in a good mood as always before going to NAMM. He worked on his van to ensure a safe trip. Also, he said we should plan to stop and pick up the rest of my furnishings and belongings from my friend,

Linda. We could use them to spruce up our little home. I agreed, hopeful again for our relationship.

We checked into an inexpensive motel on Katella Boulevard up the street from the convention center. Once we got to Anaheim, Grayson left me by myself and went to the convention early in the morning. He returned so late that he just passed out for 3 hours and got up and did it all over again. He didn't even meet me for a meal the whole time we were there. I had expected to help him in his booth at the show taking orders. I also expected to join him for social interactions but none of that happened. He just got up the first morning of the convention and went off without me and he refused to answer his phone.

I felt trapped in the motel room. I kept expecting Grayson to return and pick me up for the day. I was afraid if I even went out for coffee or some ice that I would miss his call. I was not allowed to have a cellular phone because we could only afford one. Since Jeremy was visiting his dad, I didn't have him for company either. I was bored and unhappy.

One the third morning, I noticed that Grayson had bought some cocaine as he had accidently left some behind in the room. Angry and feeling entitled, I helped myself to some of it and then used a little more. Before long the little plastic bag was empty. It was almost 12 hours before Grayson returned looking for his stash.

By then Jeremy had been returned by Alan to the motel. We were to return to Utah the following morning. Grayson was irate that I had helped myself to his cocaine and we fought. He called me horrible names and was threatening. It was 12 am and Grayson took off again. He said that if he stayed, he'd beat the crap out of me. When he returned several hours later, I pretended to be asleep in the second queen bed with Jeremy. By 4 am, reassured that there would be no further incident, I drifted off to sleep.

It had been a long night. The plan was to leave at 11 am to travel back home. I woke around 9:30 am. Jeremy had turned the TV on and was watching cartoons. I rubbed my eyes and noticed immediately that Grayson's suitcase was not in the room and neither was he.

I jumped out of bed and looked out the window to the parking lot below. The van was gone! What was this?

I called Grayson to no avail. He wasn't picking up. The skies were grey and cloudy, and a light rain had started to fall. I wanted to believe that he had gone to gas up the van or finish some last-minute business. As it got closer to check out time at 11 am my increasing anxiety and feeling of dread got stronger and stronger.

11 am passed and then it was noon. The front desk called the room asking for the keys. They said Grayson had paid the bill but that we needed to check out of the room by 1pm at the latest. It started to hit me.

It was 3 years to the day that we had met at this very same location. Grayson had packed up his belongings (with the rest of mine) and left for Utah without us. He had left us homeless in Anaheim.

I checked my pockets. I had $20. Jeremy and I each had old worn suitcases. The kind without wheels.

By 1pm the rain was coming down hard. I sat with Jeremy in the motel office until 6pm still hoping against all hope that Grayson would return and fetch us. But he didn't and the motel clerk shooed us out into the rain to fend for ourselves.

My $20 wouldn't get us a room. I looked up and down Katella and noticed a phone booth on the corner. I got some change from a convenience store and ushered Jeremy into the phone booth. I pushed our suitcases in with us and called my mom.

It was 7 days after the 1994 Northridge earthquake. When my mom answered the phone, she seemed distraught and disorganized. I tried to explain to her what had happened, but she just kept circling back to the earthquake. I begged her to come and pick me and Jeremy up, but she said she didn't know how she would get to us.

I tried to hold it together as Jeremy was in that tight space with me hearing every word. Finally, I cut to the chase. I said, "Mom, I get that there was an earthquake, but I am standing here in a phone booth with your grandson. It's pouring rain outside. What should I do?"

She seemed very far away. In a tiny frail voice, she said, "I don't know Je'net. I just don't know... I have to go now, David's calling me..."

And then she hung up.

Jeremy and I tried to get warm in the phone booth. People were walking by, tourists mostly. They looked at us with either pity or disgust, or both. Two rough looking men came up and wanted to use the phone. They started banging on the clear glass, and I was afraid they might shatter it. As the exchange became more heated, a tall scraggly woman pushed her way through the small crowd that had formed. She motioned to me to get close to the door and crack it open a bit. It was obvious to me that she was a prostitute.

She said to me, "Look honey, you can't stay here. It's not safe. You are keeping these guys from doing their business. Someone is going to call the police. Get out of there and come with me. I got a room up the street. You and your kid can stay with me tonight."

Reluctantly, but with appreciation we followed our new friend, Karen, down the street to the "Golden Forest" motel.

That night after Jeremy was asleep, I witnessed Karen and her boyfriend shoot up heroin. I had never seen that before. Although I did flashback to the past when I had played the part of a prostitute who did in the theatre production, "Homeless, a Street Opera, Life Imitating Art."

I don't know what would have happened to Jeremy and myself that night without Karen. Even though the next morning it was clear that Karen had helped herself to my belongings, even wearing my clothes right in front of me. Yet, I will be forever indebted to my untraditional agent of rescue. God sends angels in all forms to help us. I believe He sent me Karen.

Chapter 17
Daddy's Little Princess Finds Her Prince

About 6 months after I had been abandoned by Grayson, I had found a desperate rhythm. I had made the difficult but appropriate decision to allow Jeremy to stay at his paternal Grandma Margaret's house during the week while I did whatever I had to do (much of this very unpleasant)to make sure that I had a nice motel room for the two of us from Friday to Sunday. This way he could maintain a better normal than he certainly would have had with me full time. Alan had gone home to live with his mom sometime after we had moved to Utah in 1992. He had tried the cruise ship circuit playing in a jazz trio, but quickly found that this was not the life for him. He decided to go back to school to become an elementary/middle school teacher. So, I would arrange to pick Jeremy up from school on Friday and return him on Sunday afternoon.

Alan and I were not getting along. He was very hurt by how I left him, and his mother felt it was all my fault. Ending a marriage is just not what you do in the old country of Scotland. What you do is suck it up and make the best of it. She had always had a pragmatic no nonsense way about her. When Jeremy was a few months old, I struggled with feeding him. He was a lazy eater and I did all I could to get him to nurse. This included wearing a bottle of formula around my neck with a tube taped to my nipple so that he would learn that he could be satisfied from taking a breast instead of surrendering to the bottle. In her thick Scottish brogue, she said, "Ah ye poor wee watanabe, is yer mother starvin' ye te death?" She could have been a little more supportive, but I knew she wasn't trying to hurt me. It was just her way and I deeply respected her strong defense of her family.

Frankly, when I came back from Utah, I was a pretty big mess. In retrospect, I am very thankful for the way we were able to work this out. If Alan had wanted to, he probably could have fought for full custody during this time, and likely won. Technically we were still married, neither of us having the funds needed to dissolve the marriage. I had been the major breadwinner when we were together. I had the ability to make a strong case for myself even in the worst of situations. Most people were surprised to learn I was homeless when they met me in normal circumstances at school functions or the market. I would be able to clean myself up for a court appearance, but Alan lacked self-confidence and the ability to thoughtfully represent himself. I think he didn't believe he looked good enough on paper to fight for Jeremy at that time. In that way we were very much alike.

One of my visits during this time was on Mother's Day weekend. I wanted Jeremy to understand why his mom was having such a hard time. I put some thought into what to share and how. I told him to imagine that when we were upset, we could blow our sadness and our secret feelings into a balloon. If we didn't let the feelings out and talk to safe people about them the balloon would get too full and pop. Then all the feelings would just explode, and we could lose control over them. I explained that this is what happened with mommy. I had kept a lot of bad things that had happened to me inside and when there was just too much sadness in me my heart kind of exploded. I said that I was trying really hard to share my feelings now with the right safe people who could help me. I told him that things were going to get better. I had given him a little diary for Mother's Day with a Mickey Mouse on the outside. I told him this might be a good place for him to share his own feelings, both sad and happy! Later when he fell asleep, I looked in his little book. He had written, "I think my mommy's feelings are really important." Few things have ever touched me as much as those deep thoughtful words from my wise 7-year old son.

Many of the weekends I had with Jeremy consisted of watching cartoons in a motel room. By the time Friday rolled around after a week of sleeping in my car, I was exhausted and slept a good portion of our time together. Jeremy was good at keeping himself occupied with Legos, his Game Boy and cartoons. He had learned those skills from our isolation in Utah. Now when I ask him about these weekends together, he says he doesn't remember me sleeping all the time. But I think there was some denial of my true condition in his little heart so that he could still see me as strong. What mattered was that we were together. And I know he was glad we no longer had to deal with Grayson, even though we didn't talk about him.

It was Sunday afternoon on June 24th,1994, and I had just returned Jeremy to Grandma Margaret. I still had the motel room for another night because I had wanted to spend the greater portion of Sunday afternoon with my son. It was a nice hotel with an outdoor pool and a park nearby. We had kept ourselves very busy. We even celebrated the first weekend in summer and got the room that had a Jacuzzi in it so we could go swimming in the room for fun. That was a big hit!

After dropping him off, I decided to go to the park to read. At the time I was reading a book called "Bad Love," by Jonathan Kellerman who was one of my favorite authors. As I sat on a park bench balancing the hardcover book on my knees, I became aware of a man approaching. I kept an eye on him without looking up trying to act completely disinterested. I suspected he might try to solicit me, and I was not in any mood for that conversation.

The man approached me and casually said, "Hey there! You know, I have a case of that book back at my place!"

"Yes," I thought silently, "and I suppose you have some sketches to show me as well?" In return I offered up an energetic glare accompanied with a few choice words that were not lady like. I think there may even have been a gesture involved. I wanted no part of this man.

His reaction caught me by surprise. The expression on his face was so surprised! He turned beat red and appeared completely flustered. He stuttered, "Lady, I am so sorry, I really am. I work at the convention center over there and I was just working a book show. They were giving away free books and I swear I have a whole case of the one you are reading. Jonathan Kellerman, right?"

I didn't know what to make of him. I looked at him, puzzled for a moment and then broke out laughing. Laughing? I had not had a good belly laugh in such a long-time. I was completely undone by it. All the barriers I built around myself came down for a moment and I found myself sitting there on this bench talking like we had known each other for a long time. He asked me about myself.

Rather than share the story I had made up for all strangers that I met, I found myself answering his questions honestly and with candor. Everything poured out of me that afternoon. With nothing to lose, I bared my soul and my story. And this man, Patrick, took it all in. He even teared up a time or two. He didn't try and fix me. He just listened until I was done. We sat for a while in silence. Then he asked if he could buy me some dinner. Instantly my guard went back up. I wasn't mean about it this time, but I told him I was not interested. That I had a room for that night and some food back in the hotel. He offered to drive me back, but I told him I had a car and was fine. Soon enough, he went his way and I went mine. But I left feeling like I had taken such a load off my shoulders. I had popped my balloon, so to speak. It was enough to carry me back to my last night before hitting the streets again with a somewhat optimistic lift.

The next morning at 11 am there was a knock on the door of my room. I wasn't surprised by this. I always waited until the front desk shooed me out. Why would I leave before they told me? Sometimes I got away with several extra hours before I moved back into my car for the week. I opened the door expecting the cleaning staff but instead there was Patrick, the man from the park.

He stood there looking at me quietly for a moment. I could tell he was feeling emotional and

I was very confused. But he opened his mouth and said just this, "Je'net.... you just don't belong... out there..." It was hard for him to say. He actually had tears in his eyes! What was this?

He went on, "Look, I don't have much. I'm basically a working bum. I live in a tiny converted garage apartment with only one bedroom. If you are willing, I will move into the living room and you and your son, Jeremy, can have the bedroom. I swear I will be a gentleman. I won't touch you. I know that that's hard for you to believe but I am a man of my word. I just feel like I am supposed to help you get back on your feet."

He paused. I looked at him, tears in my own eyes. Should I trust this man? What made him any different from the other men who had promised to take care of me while I was homeless? Once before I allowed a man pay for a motel room for a month for me and Jeremy. Ultimately there was another price for me to pay. Merely a cost to my soul that meant nothing to me anymore. Could it hurt to give this a try? Would I be able to have Jeremy with me more than just on the weekends if I did this?

I looked at the ground and then around at my open and stuffed suitcase full of what I had left to my name, which was not much. Fighting back some tears of my own, I said softly, "Okay."

The apartment was in a row of tiny houses on an old established street in Anaheim near the Colony. One of the houses had a garage that had been converted to this modest unit. The whole thing couldn't have been more than 600 square feet. True to his word, he gave up his bedroom to me and Jeremy. Also, true to his word, he didn't try to man handle me. There was only space enough in the bedroom for a twin sized bed and I remember thinking, "Well he can't be much of a player with that bed!"

I took the bed and Jeremy slept in a sleeping bag on the floor at the foot of the bed. His little three-foot body fit perfectly in that cozy spot between the wall and the footboard. It was the tiniest apartment I had ever seen. It didn't take more than a few steps to get from one side of the living room to the other. The living room had a small loveseat sofa and a Lazy-Boy chair. Pat slept most nights in the Lazy-Boy chair and occasionally he slept on the floor. When he slept on the floor, I would literally have to step over him to get to the kitchen or to the bathroom. But there was no check out time here, and I was able to focus on more than weekend lodging. I unpacked my clothes and Jeremy's clothes in a dresser that Patrick emptied for me. We all shared the one closet in the bedroom but that was okay as none of us had much. Pat wore nothing but shorts and t-shirts and I only had the one suitcase. Jeremy's belongings fit in a small duffle bag. Alan and I started sharing Jeremy on the weekdays and split up the weekend between us. Margaret who was helpful in her quiet way, always sent Jeremy with clean clothes.

Yet it certainly wasn't all happiness and roses. For the next three years I put this poor man through hell! I was absolute about my need for independence. I had to feel in control all the time. Years later he would admit to me that he fell in love with me in the park that day, but he knew that if he shared that I would run. He was right, I would have. I was only okay with the arrangement being completely on my terms. I liked this man but was darned if I was going to let him get close to me and then hurt me. Against my will, I had started to care for Patrick, and it terrified me. So, I went out on him. I was indifferent towards him. I believe that I was cruel at times. I even stole from him.

In the bedroom closet when we arrived, Pat had a huge Sparkletts water bottle where he kept spare change. It was close to full. I am sure there was more than $1500 in that thing. And he left it in there in the bedroom closet with me! Careless man! Over the months he kept putting change in the bottle, but the level stopped rising because I was taking what I needed from it for food, alcohol, and even drugs. I never used drugs when Jeremy was around, but my heart was still a big black hole that couldn't be filled. Drinking and drugs helped numb the pain I had from being thrown away by my family. Before too long there was no money left in the bottle at all, yet he never acted like he noticed. He just kept putting his change in there every night without fail.

I made every effort to give Patrick reason to cut me loose and send me on my way. In my mind this is what all men did. I was absolutely sure that the relationship would end. I wanted the relationship to end because of something I did, not because of who I was. I came back from Utah with such low self-esteem. Inexplicably, I felt empowered when I walked the streets and controlled transactions. Obviously, this was painful for Patrick to watch but he never talked down to me or talked derogatorily about my coping mechanisms. I think he had just made up his mind to wait me out like a wild animal. On the nights that Jeremy was at his grandmother's house, we would sometimes be close and even intimate. The tenderness he had for me was unnerving and upset my balance. I was a walking time bomb.

When Jeremy was at his Grandmother's, my drug use could be bad and keep me up for days. I kept trying not to feel the pain I had inside. My entire family had turned their back on me. My mother in her state of denial refused to acknowledge the sexual abuse I had suffered. My brother had taken deliberate steps to make sure no one we knew would help me. He painted me as nothing more than a drug addict, completely discounting the resurfaced memories of abuse I had suffered by my father as a potential cause for my behavior. He had used drugs and alcohol for a time in his coping with what he had remembered but had pulled himself out of that with a 12-Step program. He felt he was working the program by refusing to offer support. He turned to food instead and gained a great deal of weight.

Time went by and one day I realized that I had not had my period for several months. In a panic I calculated back when I had had my last one and it was over 3 months before. I went to planned parenthood and found out that I was 14 weeks pregnant! I was very slim at this time and even thought I was beginning to show. I told Pat. I was so upset. I told him there was no way I could have this child and that I had used too much over the past several months and there was no way that the child would be born without problems. We made a very difficult decision to end the pregnancy. I looked with despair at the Sparkletts bottle knowing full well the money in there would have covered it. We made a very difficult call to my stepfamily for help, but they were Catholic and wouldn't hear of it. They wouldn't help us and stopped answering my calls.

Finally, we pulled together $400 and set the appointment for an abortion. I was a complete wreck this whole time. I wanted it to be over but so ashamed and upset with myself for not being more careful. The whole situation just made me want to be high even more. I wanted to reject the reality of where life had brought me. Was I to be a murderer now?

When it was all over, I sobered up. The loss of this child devastated me. It made me realize that I really wanted a family with Pat, but I felt I had screwed it up so bad by trying to make him hate me. He had stood by me through years of so many lows and nothing made him stop loving me, not even this.

The love that Patrick showed me was different than anything I had ever known because it was *unconditional.* I had never experienced someone loving me no matter what and not expecting anything in return. I came to realize and truly believe that he would always love me! Maybe it was time to love him back.

Chapter 18
Loss of Life

Choosing to end the life of a child comes with emotional scars that last a lifetime. That story remains true for both Patrick and me. The procedure itself is short and clinically sterile. During the procedure, no one wants to make eye contact. There is nothing but sorrow about the whole thing. I know that if I had it to do over, I would never make the same decision. At the time, I was just so sure that my drug use would have made this baby very sick, and I didn't believe that she or he would survive if I carried to term.

Yet, the loss of that pregnancy made me harshly aware of the significance of life, including my own. Patrick had not left my side, even after this terrible sin. It left me with an urgent need for family. For the one I had with Jeremy, the one Pat was offering me, and the one I wanted to create with him. After I recovered fully, we set about intentionally creating a life together. Our daughter, Jennifer, was born just about one year later.

We moved almost immediately into a larger apartment in Garden Grove. The larger apartment had a bedroom for Jeremy, one for us, and one for the baby we hoped to have soon. Quite a step up for us. Pat was doing well at work and I contributed what I could with part-time legitimate jobs. We didn't have much but we could pay our bills every month. We even got a dog, Charlie, a shepherd collie mixed breed with a beautiful calico colored coat and big expressive eyes.

It was the 3rd week of January 1995. The NAMM show was back in town and Patrick was working the show as a teamster. He was gone early morning to late night for several weeks setting up this large convention. It was the same show I had met Grayson at in 1991. It was almost exactly one year after he had left me on the streets.

Early one morning after Pat had left for work the phone rang. It was Grayson. My heart skipped a beat, then two, and I literally choked and grabbed my chest. I couldn't respond at first. But it didn't matter. The call was not for me, it was for him. He sounded all happy and energized and shared that he had decided to "do the right thing." He said he decided to bring back all my belongings from Utah, rather than throw them away. Grayson remarked with a laugh that he certainly could have "and should have" thrown them away. He wanted to know where he could take these things. Part of me was terrified as I held the phone away from my ear.

But the other part of me desperately wanted him to see that I had landed on my feet with someone who honestly loved me and took care of me. The apartment that we were living in was 1000 times nicer than the lopsided shack Grayson and I had last shared. I wanted him to see that. So, I agreed to let him come over and drop things off.

I wanted Pat to be home, but Grayson said he could only come that afternoon. It was raining as it was a year earlier. Jeremy was at his dad's, but I had Charlie if anything were to go wrong. Charlie could bark up a storm when a stranger came to the door. And my neighbors were close by. Grayson said he would be over around 4 pm. True to his nature he still had not shown up by 9pm that night. When he finally arrived after waiting for close to 5 hours, I had worked myself into quite a nervous state. I let him in and cringed a little when he came close to hug me, but I didn't know how to say no. Charlie growled and looked puzzled. I thought I would have the courage to tell him off and show him how well I was doing while remaining in control. Yet the minute I saw Grayson, I felt small and frightened, almost sick to my stomach. I desperately wished I had told him not to come without Pat there. Grayson looked casually around and then left out the door. He began to load things into the 3rd bedroom. I began to feel ill. I went into the restroom where I began almost immediately cramping up and feeling dizzy. There was a lot of blood in the toilet. When I stood up, I panicked. My head started spinning and I fell to the floor of the bathroom with a small pool of blood forming between my legs!

I called out to Grayson and begged him to call 911, but he just looked at me in disgust and said, "You think I am going to call the cops here and have you tell them that I have some part in this? You'll be fine." While I fell in and out of consciousness, I could hear him coming in and out of the apartment for what seemed like an hour. I was crying and asking for him to bring me the phone from the living room. Eventually, he came back to the bathroom, phone in hand. He said, "You know, I was glad to hear that you were still alive when I called you. I thought you might be dead. Looks like I was almost right. You are such a mess, Je'net, a fucking mess. You haven't changed at all. I was right to leave here without you." With that he dropped the phone far enough away from me to know I would have to crawl to reach it. He turned on his heels and walked away. Gasping for air, I struggled to the phone and dialed 911 for help. I tried to call Pat too, but had a hard time remembering his number.

In the distance I could hear sirens, and before long the EMTs were there. I asked them to call Pat for me and they said they would at the hospital, but they needed to get me there right away. I was panicked about all the blood. They covered me up and were rolling me out the door into the rain when Pat came around the corner. He finally arrived home from work. When I saw him, I felt a rush of relief and then must have passed out.

The next thing I remember was being at the hospital. I awoke terrified with someone's hands inside me feeling around. This triggered me and I started to scream and struggle. Without warning a flashback hit me full on. I was on my bed back in Ohio and my brother was there. I could see him between my legs looking up inside me with an empty bottle of soda in his hand. He was pushing it in and out of me. The etched glass, a trademark of the soft drink TAB, was scraping me and making me cramp. It hurt so much! I panicked! The nurses were grabbing for my arms and holding me down. I was hysterical and out of control. One of the medical team injected me with a needle and I fell back on the table exhausted and weak. I stared up at the ceiling in defeat.

This was my first memory of my brother's sexual abuse towards me. Up to now, I had thought that my father abused me and that my brother had been abused by him as well. But after this first memory of my brother's abuse surfaced, many others followed. These memories were mean spirited and painful. My brother's eyes were expressionless as if he were completing a science experiment on a corpse. I felt sub-human and without worth.

The doctor came in to talk to me and Pat. He asked me if I had recently had a procedure and we told him about the abortion. He said that they had apparently not completed the procedure and that there were still remnants of tissue still inside me.

I thought, "Remnants of tissue?" I imagined the worst. Was there still a baby inside me?

That's what caused the bleeding. The doctor told me I would need a DNC. Basically, that meant that I would need to go back in and have the procedure repeated. My eyes welled up with tears. I remember thinking *I would not be able to handle that again.* Just as I had growing up, I fell into a deep hole of depression and pushed away any and all feelings. I thought to myself, *I'm an expert at this. I will just drift away.*

It turned out to be just as difficult as I thought. The next few months would be overwhelming and particularly traumatizing. I knew I was being punished for the original decision and believed that I deserved everything I got.

Chapter 19
Valentine's Day

After a time of healing, Patrick and I started to intentionally try and get pregnant. I think we were both very aware that this was also our way of coping with the loss we had just experienced. We didn't talk about it much. It was too painful. We tried to look to the future and hoped that the physical trauma my body had undergone would not stand in the way of a future pregnancy. Pat had asked me to marry him and I had accepted. We wanted to expand our new family as soon as I was well enough. Marriage arrangements had to be put off for the future. My first husband, Alan, and I were still legally married. The only thing standing in the way of completing this divorce was the money to pay for it and the determination for legal custody of Jeremy. This process would take another year of mediation with the courts.

I finally felt that I was able to make a commitment to Patrick. I became pregnant in June1995, just a few months later. We were excited and I cautiously believed in the love that Pat had for me. I hoped with all my heart I could give love back as well as he so freely gave it. I still struggled with my demons but at least now I didn't try and hide it. Pat helped as much as he could. I was due in late February of 1996.

The phone rang on February 14th, Valentine's Day. Of course, it would be Patrick calling to ask if he could bring me something on his way home from work. He was working and we were planning to try and go out to eat that weekend and still no dinner plans had been made. When I picked up the phone, I was shocked to hear Grayson's voice on the phone. He sounded jovial, maybe high, and acted as if the last time we saw each other had never happened. This phone call hit me hard and to the core. My hands were shaking as I put the phone back in its cradle. I started to hyperventilate.

I called Pat and he rushed home to me. He took me to the hospital, and I went into early labor. I was far enough along that this would not hurt the baby. As I tried to pull myself into the wonder of delivery, I couldn't help cursing this man who had invaded so much of my life. It seemed like it would never end. I allowed myself to accept an epidural this time. When Jeremy had been born, I endured over 21 hours of hard labor with no pain medication. In the end, I had an emergency Cesarean section because his heart rate was struggling. Jeremy's umbilical cord had been wrapped around his shoulder, which had kept him from slipping into the birth canal. I kept fixating on that. I asked the nurse over and over if Jennifer was ok? Jennifer was born after seven hours of labor! During the birthing process, I was so distraught and clearly unstable that after Jennifer was born, a county worker came to talk to me. They ran tests to determine my sobriety. They talked to me about my extreme reactions to the medical team as they delivered the baby. Apparently, I had been triggered and so emotional that they had to sedate me. They counseled me to get a psychiatric evaluation for Jennifer's sake. They opened an informal case and set me up with services at UCI. I was terrified they might take Jen. The nurse assured me that if I sought out treatment, the case would be closed in 6 months.

When we got home and settled in with our newborn, I had a lot of soul searching to do. I blamed myself for letting my past haunt me over and over. This should be nothing but a happy time. Yet, my hormones were off the chart and I knew deep inside that I needed help.

I was referred to a lady that would watch Jennifer when I needed to keep my appointments with mental health. Her name was Marsha. Marsha would change my life forever.

Chapter 20
On My Knees

For six months after Jennifer was born, I went to a therapy session for an hour each week. I was connected to a wonderful lady named Marsha who would watch my baby girl while I went to the session. She was a small slight figured woman with straight blonde hair and a quick smile. I was really impressed with how she ran her home with so many children running around. It seems there was always somebody running in the front door and somebody else running out the back door. She had five children of her own and watched another three or four on a regular basis. It was the kind of house I always wished I had grown up in. Her house had a lot of positive energy, always something happening, even if that included some firm words and strict discipline. The house smelled of freshly baking cookies, pies and sometimes even fresh bread. And there was always a plan in place to prepare for the evening meal with all the kids lending a hand.

Marsha was sweet and encouraging. I could tell that she truly loved Jennifer. Early on she invited me to church with her, but I didn't want anything to do with that. What impressed me about the situation was that she didn't push when I said no. At that time, I still could not imagine myself putting my trust in someone other than Patrick. I still didn't believe fully that our relationship wouldn't end.

At this point in my life, I thought I had it all back together. I had a husband and a baby. Also, Alan and I had finally gotten divorced. We each had equal and shared custody of Jeremy. We were all together living in a townhome in Orange. Pat and I had one bedroom and the kids shared the other bedroom.

Yet, I was still severely depressed. I struggled with my sobriety off and on. Some days I would be good and other days I would feel like I had fallen back into the depths of my despair. I wondered if I would ever feel completely safe and happy.

I had tried to go back to work several times. I usually interviewed very well and got a position in management. But before long the voices in my head would start to remind me that I was not worthy. I worried that people would know I was just faking my way through the job and I was inadequate. I would begin to doubt myself and come in late to work or call in sick so they would have a reason to fire me. Eventually, I filed for disability because of my trauma and PTSD. I was awarded Social Security benefits. In my head, I heard the words, "You're so screwed up the government will pay you to stay home."

So, I went to therapy, filled my days with a lot of endless and mindless TV, and for a solid year I could not understand why I felt so damn miserable. What was wrong with me?

During that era, Marsha would gently but consistently bring up the subject of this meeting at her church. She had backed off from inviting me to service, but she did encourage me to attend a women's meeting on Wednesday nights. She told me, "It's not really like going to church, it's more of a gathering to talk about ourselves and our challenges. You will feel right at home, I promise you. This group is meant for you."

Honestly, she looked so happy when she talked about the group and never pushed too hard. So, one afternoon when I was particularly struggling with my sobriety, I called Marsha and asked her when that meeting started. As it turned out, I was calling on Wednesday, and the meeting was that night. I told her I would consider coming and hung up the phone.

I knew I didn't want to use drugs or alcohol that night. I knew that the way I was feeling I probably would if I stayed home. So, I decided that I would go to this church meeting and just observe.

Nothing prepared me for the love and acceptance that was in that room that night. The group was called Joy Renewed. Most of women there had a history of abuse, trauma, jail, prison, or a criminal record. At first, I was put off, as clearly my friend Marsha had seen me as a good fit for this motley crew. I wanted to feel superior to them but in my heart, I knew I was just like them. They welcomed me with smiles and hugs.

The group was led by a sweet little old English lady named Chaplin Patricia Nesbit and her husband, Bob. They both lead ministry teams into the jails and invited women that they met there to join this group once they were released. It was clear that Chaplin Pat had a pure heart and nothing about her was judgmental. She told beautiful, rich and descriptive stories about her life in England during the war. Clearly, she loved sharing the wisdom from the Bible and made the scriptures come alive. I didn't know anything about the Bible, but I wasn't the only one there who didn't. That helped a lot.

Ninety minutes later, Chaplain Pat led an altar call. She invited anyone who did not know the Lord to come forward. I told her that I didn't know if I could say the prayer when I didn't know if I could believe in Jesus. She asked me if I was willing to consider the possibility that Jesus was the son of God, that God was real and had a purpose for me and a purpose for my life. She told me the story about only needing faith the size of a mustard seed. And then she showed me a picture of a Mustard seed. It was so tiny… I told her I was willing to consider the possibility that there might be a God, that he might be real, and that I had a sincere desire to know Him if He was… *real.*

And then I was down on my knees reciting the sinner's prayer. It was November 11, 1998.

Chapter 21
A Walk in Forgiveness

Within the first several months after I got saved, God seemed to be impressing something on my heart. I still felt angry that my family had turned their backs on me when my memories of abuse surfaced and when I was homeless. Anger and resentment ate away at my new-found joy. I talked about it in our group on Wednesday nights and Chaplin Pat responded by giving a message regarding forgiveness. She taught me that forgiveness doesn't have to be for the other person. In fact, forgiveness is often more important for the one who is doing the forgiving than the one who needs to be forgiven. I began to work on this part of my journey.

I was astonished that it was comparatively easy to forgive my father for what he had done to me. His abuse had happened long ago. Of course, he had been dead for 26 years by this time. I know it may be difficult for the reader to understand but I did not feel as victimized by him as I did by my mother and my brother. It was my mother who stood on the sideline, who could have protected me and didn't. She never stood with me on my side. And it was my brother who chose to continue to abuse me well after my father had passed away. He was 16 by that time and certainly had a choice. Hard to imagine that he didn't know that having sexual relations with his sister was wrong. He was the one who would come to my room at night, not the other way around. Both mom and Jack made conscious decisions not to help me when I was strung out, suicidal and homeless. They turned me away when I desperately needed help. This was not the time for Tough Love. I imagine it was easier for them to believe that I was just a lost soul who had made very bad choices for myself and deserved what I got. In fact, my choices had been taken away from me for a very long time and it was the total lack of unconditional love in our family that did the most damage. My dad included, all three of them taught me in their own way that I needed to earn their love, one way or another. I could never measure up to their expectations. They never just loved me for who I was.

Yet God was doing this work in me. So, I set out to find my mother. I had not spoken to her for a couple of years. The last time was from a phone booth in Anaheim on the night Grayson had abandoned me and Jeremy. I knew she was ill and that my stepfamily had put her in a care facility, but I didn't know where. I was discouraged to find out that she was all the way out in Simi Valley in a skilled nursing center. Patrick and I shared just one vehicle and he used it daily for work. So, I packed up the kids and traveled by train to see my mother. Jeremy was 11 or 12 and Jennifer was just under two years old. It was a moderately long journey with the two kids in tow. Once we got to the train station, we still had to walk to the nursing home a half mile away.

Mom was in a pretty bad state. The first time we saw her I was shocked to see how much she had declined. She was only 66 years old, but she was curled up into a fetal position being fed through a G-tube inserted into her stomach. Her eyes were vacant and stared off into space. She did not appear to be present in the room at all but stuck in her own sad reality. She seemed to be worried or frightened. Laying on her side she rocked back-and-forth alternatively moaning and making mewing sounds of distress. My heart went out to her. It was almost like looking into a mirror. I saw the hopelessness and pain in her expression… I knew it all too well. I approached her bed and spoke softly to her.

"Hi, mom…It's me, Je'net." For a moment, I thought she responded. She uttered a sound that had it been a word might have been, "What?"

"It's me, mom. It's your daughter, Je'net. I am here with Jeremy. And this is our daughter, Jennifer. You haven't met her yet."

She turned her head to one side and then the other. Like she was trying to find something. She appeared puzzled and then I watched as she appeared to see something else in the room. She seemed to panic and started to rock back and forth again, distressed.

I thought, "Oh gosh, what have I brought the kids out to see?" I considered sending them out of the room but set them up in a corner with a handheld Gameboy instead. I handed Jennifer a fruit roll up and she settled in next to her brother.

I continued to try and talk to her, but she wouldn't respond. Then I had a thought. Maybe she would respond if I sang quietly to her. I started with Amazing Grace. She stopped rocking and seemed to be listening to me from somewhere deep inside her consciousness. I kept singing hymns I had learned in church. This went on for almost 30 minutes. I decided to sing one more and then say our goodbyes.

Something remarkable was about to happen. I had run out of hymns and had started to sing ballads from some of the musicals I knew. I remembered one of her favorites was "Someone to Watch Over Me," a Gershwin classic. I began to sing this for her. These are the lyrics of the song:

There's a somebody I'm longing to see

I hope that he turns out to be,

someone to watch over me

I'm a little lamb who's lost in the wood,

I know I should, always be good

To one who'll watch over me.

Although he may not be the man some girls think of as handsome,

To my heart, he carries the key

Won't you tell him please to put on some speed?

Follow my lead, Oh, how I need…

Someone to watch over me"

As I began the song, Dorothy seemed to come into the room and be present. She opened her eyes and seemed to see me. She was peaceful and I even thought I detected a small smile. As I finished the song singing the title phrase, she suddenly became alert and locked her eyes with mine.

Startled, I said, "What is it mom?" She looked me dead on. I was sure she wanted to tell me something but couldn't find the motor skills to do so. The look in her eyes was urgent. She struggled but somehow found her voice. It looked like it took all the energy she had. She opened her mouth and said with great difficulty just one word, "GOD."

She said it in such a way and with such desperation that I literally took two steps back and just looked at her. Was she asking God to watch over her? What was I supposed to do with this statement? I was speechless and unable to continue singing. I just hugged her as she slipped away again. One moment she was there, and the next moment she had disappeared back to wherever her soul was being tortured. She fell asleep and was quiet.

That night, I went back to my Saint of a husband, Patrick, this incredible man who had already done his part by rescuing me and my son from the streets and showing us great kindness. I asked, or rather begged, him to allow me to bring my mother home and take care of her. Like the man he is, he didn't even pause for a moment. He simply said, "Of course we can."

Chapter 22
Photographs

Je'net's parents, Jerry and Dorothy.

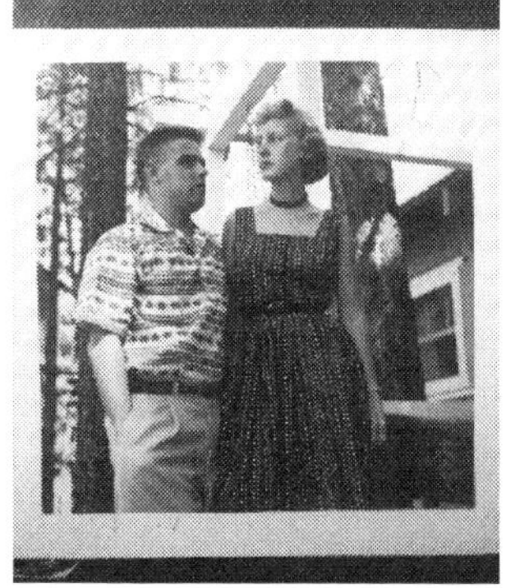

Je'net's Great Grandmother Louise Raife.

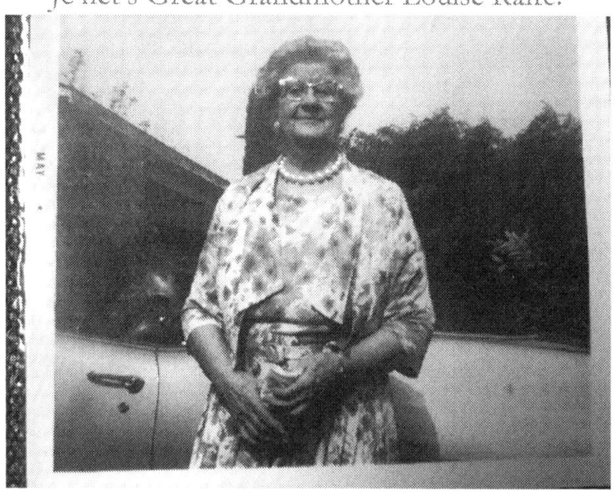

Je'net's mother, Dorothy Doran, from her days at Paramount Studios.

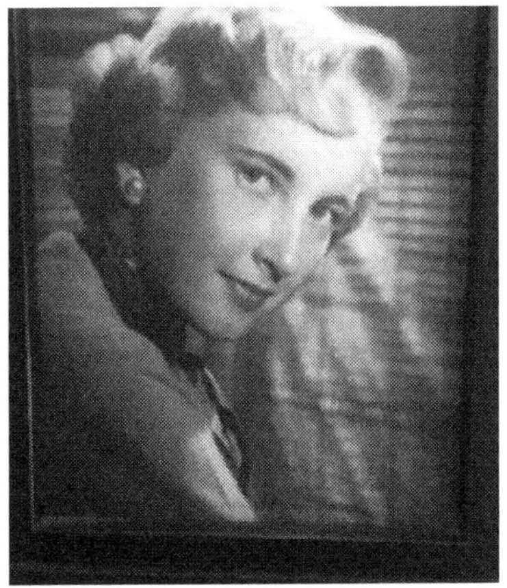

Je'net's theatrical headshot.

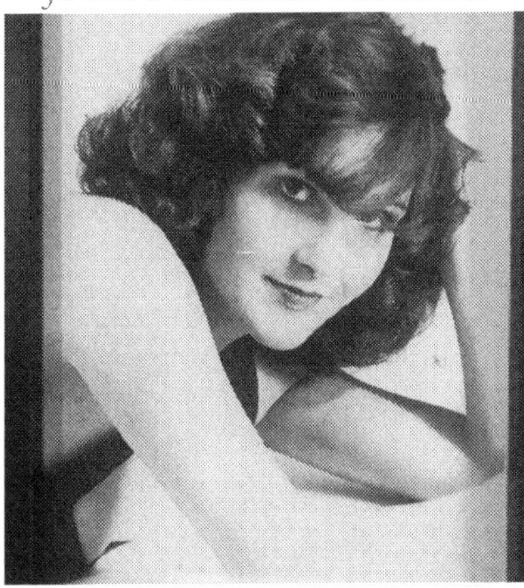

Je'net in Cabaret.

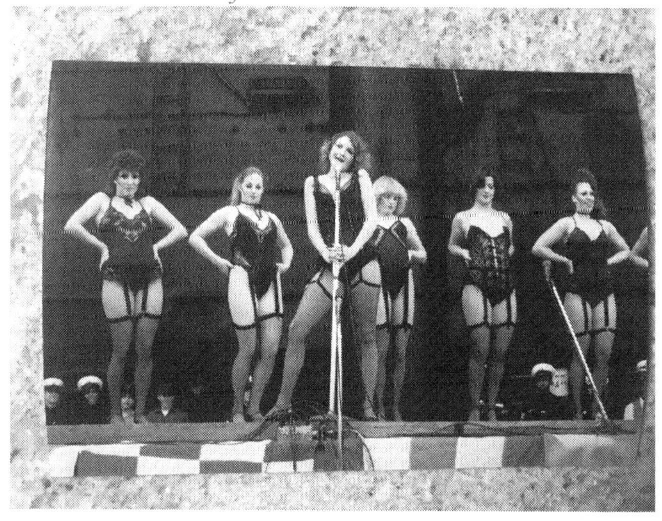

Cabaret review.

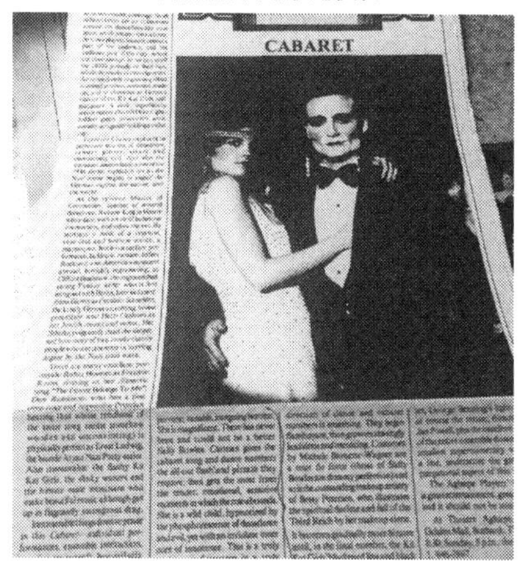

CABARET

Bob Gregory Show with Love.

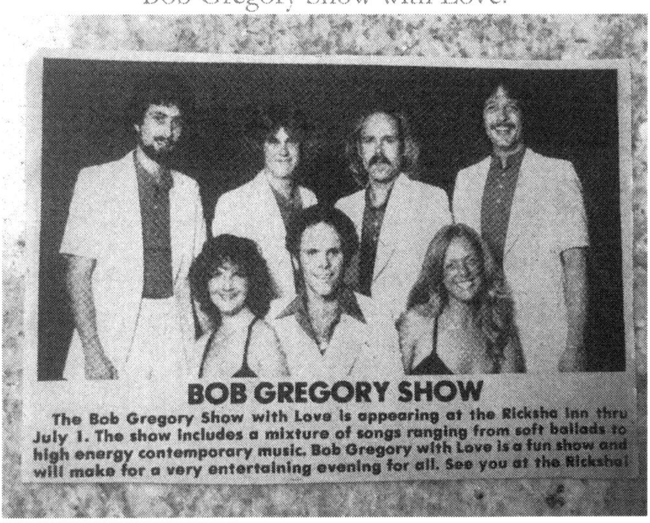

BOB GREGORY SHOW

The Bob Gregory Show with Love is appearing at the Ricksha Inn thru July 1. The show includes a mixture of songs ranging from soft ballads to high energy contemporary music. Bob Gregory with Love is a fun show and will make for a very entertaining evening for all. See you at the Ricksha!

Je'net's and Patrick's wedding picture.

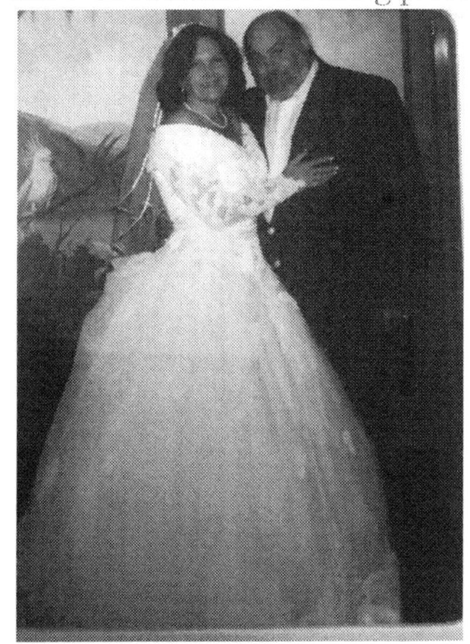

Je'net with her son, Jeremy, on her wedding day.

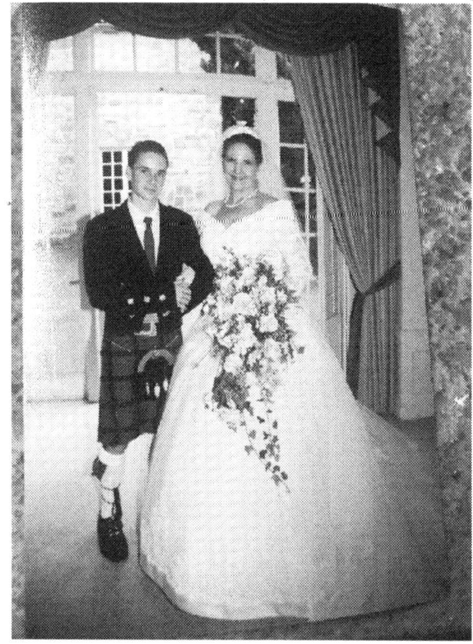

Je'net and her beloved Chaplain Patricia Nesbit.

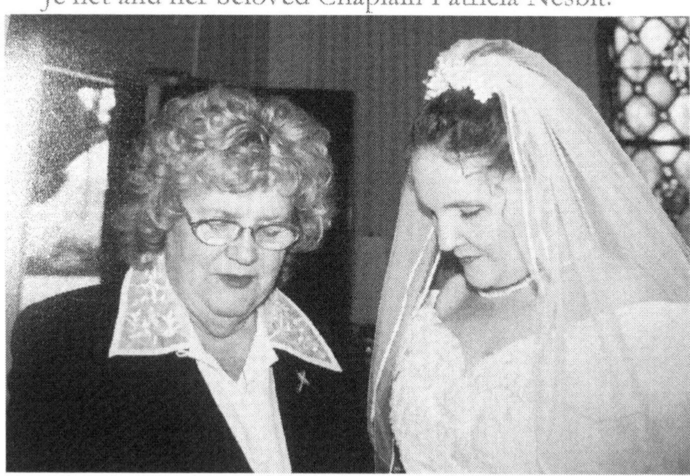

Our family on Jeremy's graduation day from the Police Academy

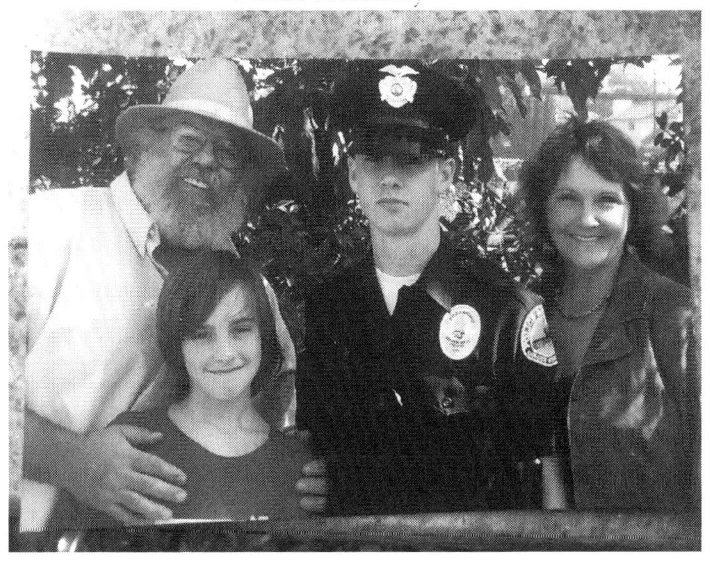

Jennifer and Vivian

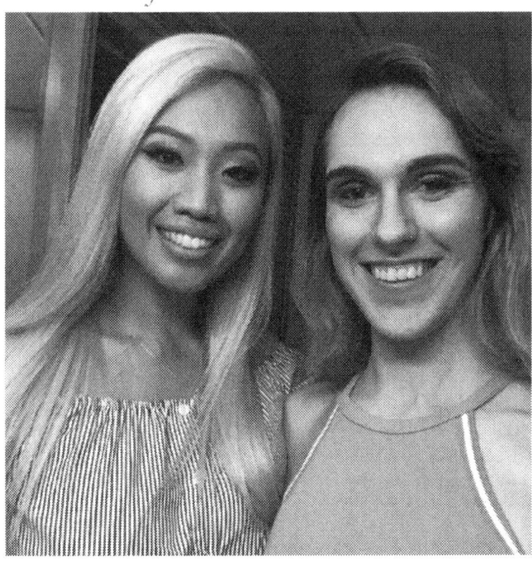

Jerry's Painting.

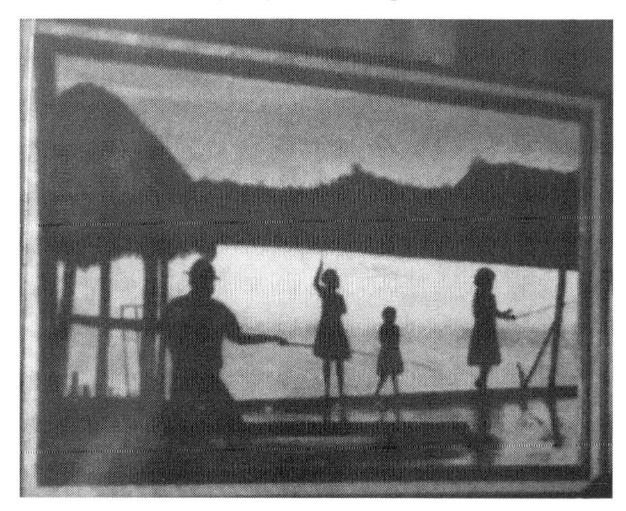

Je'net gets baptized.

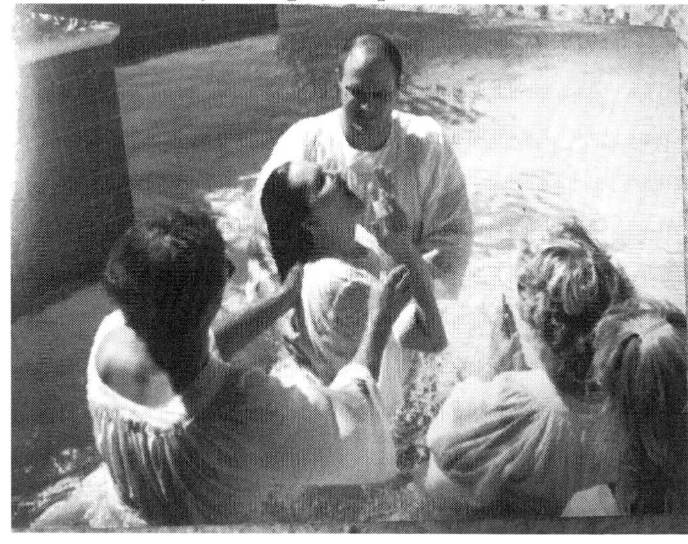

Chapter 23
"There's No Place Like Home"

I negotiated with my stepfamily. They seemed very eager to get my mother off their hands, and their checkbooks. The treatment that mom was getting at the nursing home was running up bills in the thousands and thousands every month. Yet, her overall health was stable, and she was not declining. It seemed that she could last quite a long time in this state at a huge expense to my stepfather. I told my stepfamily that I was willing to care for my mom but would need to move to a place with a downstairs bedroom to do so. Eventually, it was decided that they would pay whatever our rent not to exceed $1500 in exchange for taking care of mom. All other expenses would be our personal responsibility if not covered under medical insurance. Naively, I agreed. I did not realize how much diapers and prescriptions alone would cut into this allowance. Nevertheless, we never looked back.

I started to look for an appropriate apartment. There were ads in the paper that I followed up on but either the bedrooms were all upstairs or there was no handicap access. On a whim, I followed a For Rent sign into a Garden Grove neighborhood of single-family residential homes. I had not even considered this believing it would be too expensive. So, I was surprised when I rolled up on a ranch style one story home with beautiful palm trees in front. The sign said the monthly rental would be $1495! I knocked on the door and the current tenants told me that the home would be shown on Saturday at noon. From the door I could see an almost Big Bear Cabin looking living room with homey furnishings. And I could see through the back window that there was a pool! It looked so inviting! I couldn't believe my luck.

I went home and told Pat about the house I had found and showed him why the cheaper apartments had not been a fit. We decided we would take the kids out to breakfast in the morning and be at the house promptly at 12:00 pm.

That evening when the kids were in bed, I turned on the TV and found myself watching a Hallmark film about a woman whose mother had Alzheimer's. I thought what a coincidence! The mother in this story could still talk and walk, but she could not remember her own daughter's name or anyone else's. To the dismay of her daughter, she would get confused and tearful and wander off in the neighborhood. Yet the daughter showed her mother unlimited devotion and love. Her prayer was to hear her mother call her by name correctly just once. As I watched this movie, which seemed to rather miraculously tie to my own situation, I became weepy more than once. Pat was watching a baseball game upstairs but came down a few times to check on me. He'd ask if I was okay? When tearfully I assured him that I was okay he would head back upstairs as he looked at me over his shoulder.

As the movie came close to the end the mom finally called the daughter by her given name, and that was it for me. I was flat out balling by this time and Pat came to the couch and sat with his arms around me. He comforted me as I got it all out. The music swelled and the movie ended. Then something happened I have never seen before or since. The Reverend Franklin Graham came on the screen and gave an altar call. When did this ever happen on TV? Both Pat and I gave our attention to what he was saying. We listened intently to his impassioned call to give one's life over to a loving God who could do ALL things. Sitting in our living room, our hearts were softened and my wonderful husband, Patrick, gave his life to The Lord and was saved. We would journey into this next chapter of our lives equally yoked together and new creations in Christ!

The next day we arrived at the rental property precisely at noon. To my surprise and chagrin, there were at least 20 people in the driveway and more cars were still pulling up! My heart sank. How would we stack up against this competition? Immediately I wished that I had put on a church dress instead of my jeans and that Patrick's ponytail was tucked up in his hat. Were the kids' clothes clean?

I jumped into action and went into my best sales pitch. I persistently shared our story with the property manager. Finally, he took me by the shoulders, looked me in the eye, and said kindly but firmly, "Look, lady, I could love you like my own mother, but if the numbers aren't there, I can't rent to you!"

He handed me a rental application and walked off to talk to another family. I filled out the paperwork in my best handwriting, but I knew the facts. While Patrick made a good living *when* he worked, he had weeks of missing paychecks when he wasn't. The application required his last 3 paychecks and he had not worked two of the three prior weeks. Things did not look good for us. We turned in the application and walked back to our car. During the walk back to the car, I remember saying to myself (for the first time) a phrase I had heard in church, "Let go and let God." That was all I could do.

The next day I said a prayer in church for the right house to present itself and was back in the newspaper ads looking for other possible rentals.

A week later we heard from the property manager. His voice sounded a little bewildered when he said, "I'm not quite sure why I am doing this, or why the owner said yes to your application, but the house is yours!"

I think I screamed a little. Patrick came running down the stairs with an urgency. He cried out, "What's wrong???" With my voice a little shaky, I said, "Honey, we got the house, WE GOT THE HOUSE!!"

Six weeks later with a little extra help from my stepdad on the security deposit and his signature as a co-signer, we moved into the beautiful house on Paloma Avenue. We began the next chapter of our lives, taking care of Dorothy.

Two weeks after Patrick, the kids and I had moved in, we welcomed Dorothy home. The house had four bedrooms and a den. There was one for each of the kids who were beyond thrilled as they had been sharing a room. Children with an age-gap of a decade had very different ideas about how to decorate. Star Wars, the chosen theme in one room and SpongeBob in the other. Not to mention they were both excited to have a pool in their own backyard!

We gave mom the master bedroom which was slightly larger and sunny. She had her own bathroom for privacy. Although she could not walk, the shower was a step in and large enough to accommodate her shower chair. Patrick would learn to carry her in there so that I could bathe her. The wheelchair miraculously made the turn off the hallway and into her bedroom if you maneuvered the chair just so.

Off the spacious living room to one side was a large sun porch the perfect size for a stand-up piano and an office. Directly across from that were accordion doors to what became Pat's and my bedroom. The room itself was the smallest of the four with barely enough room for our bed and one dresser. Our room had a very small closet. Most of my clothes would live in mom's room and Patrick's clothes were folded in the drawers. Patrick routinely had to crawl over me to get to his side of the bed. When we were not looking for privacy, I would open the accordion doors to the living room. I could see all that space in front of me across the living room and into the porch, which put my anxiety about closed spaces to rest. I couldn't believe this whole house was ours to live in!

The lot was huge as well, nearly 10,000 square feet. The back yard had an enormous jumbo-sized pool and covered patio. It was perfect and much nicer than anything I ever dreamed we would find.

Mom seemed to be happy with her new situation, even if she could not tell us so in her own words. She seemed to perk up almost immediately. We would bring her out into the living room several times a day for meals and to watch TV with us. Pat would sometimes keep her company in her room and hold her hand as he watched a ball game. When he did, he would ask her over again, "Dorothy, can you say Pat?"

She would look at him confused and say nothing until one afternoon when Pat was particularly intent on trying to teach her his name. Once again, he asked her, "Dorothy, can you say Pat? Say Pat, Dorothy!"

She eyeballed him questionably, opened her mouth to speak and said clearly, "George….?"

Pat laughed and patted her hand, "That's good enough for me, Dorothy. George it is!"

Just six weeks later we celebrated Thanksgiving. Mom was sitting at the dining room table with us for this festive meal. Incredibly, unassisted she was able to pick up a few pieces of her dinner with her own hands and put them in her mouth. She had come so far from the curled-up creature I had visited in the nursing home. It seemed indeed to be a miracle, and it was happening right in front of us!

We had met the owners of the home when we first moved in. They were Christians! Our landlords were a mother and daughter team who had owned the home for over a decade. When they came to meet us, they prayed over my mom and laid hands on her. They were so gentle and so kind. They were another sign that God was meeting us on our journey.

We were devastated when we received word two years later that the owners had plans to sell the house and move out of state. Surely there was no way we could afford to buy this home! My stepdad declined to help us. Almost unheard of, the owners offered to carry the loan for us. They had hoped that we would be the buyers. Remarkably, the asking price was only $10,000 more than they had paid for the house a decade before!

But as we delved into the paperwork necessary to get approved for the loan, we discovered a $6,000 tax lien against Patrick that we didn't know about. This was a deal breaker for the owner willing to carry the mortgage contract. If we defaulted on the loan, the IRS would be first in line to take the property. Our hopes crashed. We had all the paperwork about the lien, and the outlook seemed dismal. We talked together about making one last ditch effort to try and negotiate a deal to pay it off in small payments and get the lien dismissed. But would it be in time? Would the owners wait?

We went to the IRS office and put our names and the document number on the sign-in sheet. We waited for close to 2 hours to be seen. Finally, I went up to the desk to inquire why it was taking so long. The lady at the counter told me she would check and be right back. About 15 minutes later she returned and motioned for Patrick and me to come forward.

She said, "Look, folks, I don't know why you're here. I can't find any lien on either of your social security numbers. There is just nothing here. Are you sure you have a lien?"

Miraculously, there was now no record of any tax lien! It was as if it had just disappeared! Could God even influence the Feds?

A few weeks later we signed the papers to buy our first home. It was November 11, 2000. That evening I went to my regular weekly home bible study. Promptly at 7 pm I walked in the door and was greeted with a rousing chorus of, "Happy Birthday!" With all that was going on, I had forgotten that it was the second anniversary of the day I had been saved. Exactly two years before I had entered church for the first time and fallen to my knees before the Lord.

It was as if God was telling me that I would never be homeless again. But, at the same time, I knew it had nothing to do with the four walls and ceiling of our physical home. He was clearly telling me I would always have a home with Him. Forever!

Chapter 24
Finding My Voice

What I knew for sure was that I needed a God who would stand in the middle of the street, stomp His feet and wave His arms so that I could see Him and be sure he was real. A high expectation from someone who had not spent a life in any kind of service to Him. But God knew I needed Him to meet me where I was, and He never let me down.

I have not sung a single lyric since I had performed in, "Homeless –A Street Opera." It was almost as if I was afraid of what else might come up for me if I allowed myself to open my mouth and perform again. Yet, it was the music that I began to hear at church that rekindled my musical spirit. I loved the songs. They were easy to learn. In a simple and beautiful way, the hymns helped me to understand scripture. I was amazed at how much of the sacred music that I learned was connected to verses in the Bible. These holy songs went along with reading and hearing the sermons at Sunday service. I found myself listening to Christian music in my car and naturally singing along. It happened very organically, not like I had intentionally decided to try and sing again. I was just singing again. People in the pews around me began to turn to me and complement my voice and the harmonies that came so quickly to me.

Someone suggested I should sing a solo in church. Ever the performer this idea intrigued me, but it also frightened me. On one hand, I worried if I still had the instrument I used to. But on the other hand, I felt that I deeply needed to share the emotions I felt when I worshipped God. I Hoped the fellowship at church would see less of my broken self if I could bring them along on a musical journey closer to His Spirit. I will never forget the first song that I sang in church. The song was called, "Jesus Doesn't Care What You've Done Before." I thought, how appropriate!

I had purchased this song from the Christian bookstore on tape. The song was set in three different keys: Low, medium and high. I had agonized over which range to sing this song. I was always most comfortable in my lower range, belting out a song to the back of the house. But this song had a gentle and almost angelic spirit about it. I asked the tech guys to play this song in the medium range. I was seriously nervous about my first public performance in 5yrs. When I was handed the microphone, I shared with the church briefly that I had recently been homeless, discouraged and broken. I shared with the congregation that the last time I had sung a song, it had brought up something so painful that I didn't think I would ever sing again. I went on to explain that the love of Jesus had encouraged me to sing and make a joyful noise unto Him.

When the music began, I immediately noticed that the song was being played in the high range and I was a bit panicked about hitting some of the high notes that were coming. But I relaxed into the story behind the song and it came out of my heart and my soul. I had a hard time not crying as the phrases depicted a loving Jesus who would overlook the sins of His children, no matter how big they were or how ugly. I still struggled to believe that God could forgive me for everything I had done, so the message of this song was very close and emotional for me.

It was for the congregation as well. I noticed many congregants weeping with me and my group from Joy Renewed were right up front sending me their prayers and support. Several people came up to me afterwards. They shared with me that the song had touched them deeply and encouraged me to continue to sing.

Sometime afterward, Marsha's husband who led a ministry team into the local jails in Orange County, asked me if I would be interested in singing special music for the jail ministry team called, Gleaners. He provided me with an application so that I could get my clearance to join them. A background check would be completed for me to be able to serve.

The form was green and the shape of an oversized index card. There was a small box on the back of the form. In that small box, I was to write any and all infractions of the law or interactions that I may have had with the police in my lifetime. I had been cautioned to be completely honest and thorough with what I put in this box. Any omission would likely result in my disqualification. I remember writing very small tiny letters so that I could fit all my indiscretions into this box. My accounting overflowed into the minimal area around it as well. I was prepared for it to take six months to a year to be completely investigated. Also, I had also been told that people with my kind of history could flat out be denied. I turned it in and hoped for the best.

Ten days later my family was scheduled to be baptized at a private home located in the hot and dry hills of Corona. We had prayed about it and had decided to bring my mother along for baptism. I remember her looking very agitated and trying to swat away the water as the pastor prayed over her as she sat in her wheelchair. The kids were both trying not to laugh. Jeremy and Jennifer were baptized in the pool with me. Patrick stayed back because he had been baptized as a child in Missouri. Years later he would be baptized anew too.

When we got home that afternoon, I noticed the blinking red light on the answering machine. I pushed playback and was astonished to hear the message. It was from Officer Dominic Mejica, the man in charge of background checks and clearance for the jail ministry teams. The message was short and concise. He informed me that I had been cleared to participate on the jail ministry team. He instructed me to call a number to schedule a time to come down and get my picture taken for my badge! I remember thinking that was so incredible considering everything I had shared on my application. It was like a gift for my baptism day. God showed me His way forward.

From thc first day I entered Santa Ana Women's Jail, I knew I was where God wanted me to be. I struggled for years to get sober for myself, for others and even for my own family. Yet the day I stood in front of all those incarcerated women for the first time, women who were experiencing the same challenges I knew so intimately myself, I knew I would never be lured back into using drugs to deal with my problems. God gave a calling to me. God wanted me to share my story with the gift of music that He had given me to those who were still in chains.

In the early days of my visits, it was quite apparent to the inmates that I was the "testimony" part of the church service. I came along with the "church ladies" and filled the role of the past offender who made good and came out a survivor. I shared from my heart and with raw reality. I'd win them over with my stories of being on the street and suffering from addiction. Then I would sing and the surprise on the inmates' faces was quite apparent. The former drug addict can sing.

I am not sure exactly when this happened, but one day I realized that my role had flipped. I would sing and lead worship. The Chaplain would give the message, and then I would share stories about my past. There was still surprise on the inmates' faces, but now because they saw me as one of the "church ladies!" My transformation was coming full circle.

Ten years later when I would renew my badge for the fifth time, I asked Dominic if he would pull my original application out and let me see it. I told him that I had always thought I was approved very quickly considering my background. I couldn't remember how long I waited to receive approval, but I had a friend who tried at the same time and never received approval.

Everything was still in hardcopy and Dominic had no trouble pulling that old green index card from the filing cabinet behind him. I remember him looking at the card and staring at it for a long minute. He nudged the officer next to him and asked her to look at it as well. Her expression also seemed puzzled.

I asked, "What is it, Dominic?"

He passed the card over to me and said, "I don't know how this happened Je'net, but your application was approved without investigation. It doesn't look like we ever did a background check on you at all! Look, it was marked approved the day we received it...and the stamp is right over the criminal history section that you filled out... I don't understand how this could have happened!"

I do.

Chapter 25
I Love You Too, Sweetheart

Taking care of a very sick parent has its own set of very personal challenges. Because Dorothy was bed bound, unlike many dementia caretakers, we did not have to worry about her wandering off into the neighborhood. Yet, the immobility that my mom experienced was imposed on her after a fall that broke her hip. Whoever made medical decisions for my mom at that time made the choice not to try and rehabilitate her, even though she was only in her early sixties. She never received any physical therapy. They did not replace her hip or follow up on care that would have helped her walk again. She was transferred at that time from a residential facility to a skilled nursing home.

I researched the care that was available for Dorothy and found that she did qualify for physical therapy, so I arranged for in home care. The physical therapist that came out to see my mom was named Shama. Shama was a gentle but firm woman from India that worked miracles. Within 6 months my mother regained her mobility and walked for the first time in 4 years! She would never walk again without assistance. It broke my heart to know that if she had physical therapy earlier on, she may have never lost this essential life-enhancing ability.

My mother's husband, David, only visited my mother twice during the 5 years we cared for her, and my brother visited her only once. It saddened me that another woman in my family was left behind because her situation was more than anyone wanted to handle.

Caring for mom was not easy. Every meal took nearly an hour for her to process. Although she had regained some use of her hands, she could not hold onto anything, nor did she have the fine motor skills necessary to hold a fork or spoon and bring it up to her mouth. She could hold on to a piece of toast but little else. Toast was too dry for her to swallow without close attention. Her favorite meal consisted of oatmeal with yogurt and bananas crushed up in it. She and I would sit in the dining room while I patiently gave her one spoonful after the other. Often, I encouraged her to chew and swallow because she would just forget what came next. It would typically take me 45 minutes to get a whole meal into her.

I came to understand why she had lost so much weight in the nursing home. I had watched them feed her while she sat around the table with 4 others. One technician would feed all 5 of them. If the patient turned away from the food or wasn't responsive, they just lost that turn. About 20 minutes was allotted to feed all 5 of them. No wonder mom didn't thrive! It was way easier to insert a tube into her stomach and push nutrients into her that way. Otherwise, she would have starved to death.

We had a choice to remove the G-tube when mom came home but ultimately decided to keep it in place because we needed to make sure mom got enough fluids all day long. She wasn't very good about swallowing clear liquids. If there was something in her mouth that didn't have texture to it, she would just open her mouth and the water would end up in her lap. It was the right decision to make, as later her ability to eat would decrease.

Mom would be physically present with us but not mentally most of the time. She would sit and stare into space with her head turning slightly from side to side. She would make noises like she was talking but no words would come out. She just mumbled. Sometimes she would react to one of our dogs barking by saying, "ruff ruff!"

But there were times when she would stir up from deep inside and a sentence would escape! Once when the dogs were being particularly friendly and nuzzling her hand for a head rub, she looked down at them slightly annoyed and said clear as day, "Oh, go to bed!" On those days we would announce, "Grandma's in the room!"

One afternoon Pastor Millie came by to visit. While I fed mom, I visited with Millie and when I finally finished, she kneeled at mom's side. She took her hand gently and said, "I'm going to pray over you now, Dorothy. Would that be all right?"

My mom focused and was suddenly present in the room with us. She looked down at Millie and said with sincere concern, "But I don't know how!"

Pastor Millie didn't skip a beat. She said, "Well now, Dorothy, it would be a privilege to show you."

While caring for mom was rewarding, it was also relentless. We really could not leave her for any substantial amount of time. I felt safe walking up to King of Kings Lutheran School to pick up Jennifer from Kindergarten but that only took about 20 minutes round trip. Even though Mom could not get out of bed, leaving her for an hour was a rare occurrence. It was taxing on the whole family as we were very limited on what we could do as a family without her. We took her with us to church and it was touching to see her hand creep up into the air on its own as if in worship. She only did this in church. It gave me great comfort to have this affirmation that she was having internal conversations with Jesus. Yet, the 90 minutes at church was about all she could handle. Going out to eat after church was rare.

We were blessed to be supported by a group called, Orange County Caregivers. They had a respite program that would provide free hours of respite to professional caregivers. Our family qualified for this free service, but the waiting list was long. We waited almost 3 years to reach the top of the list. When we reached the top of the list it was life changing. Although some friends from church would occasionally come to stay with mom so we could attend school events and the like, they always felt nervous given my mom's extreme frailty. Not too many were comfortable changing an adult diaper, so we'd have to make plans around mom's hygiene schedule. When OC Caregivers helped us with in-home care and respite, we finally were able to take a trip to Disneyland with the kids. What a celebration we had that day!

One day Pat was transferring mom from the bed to the chair and partially lost his grip on her. She sprained a knee and she was in a lot of pain. Her doctor prescribed pain medications to help her be comfortable. While the pain medication worked for her knee, it would also ultimately take my mom from us.

She slipped away from us a little each day after this. When we tried to lessen the pain meds, she would appear to be in agony. We chose to keep her comfortable, believing it would only take a few weeks for her to heal.

Not long after, Jennifer performed in her first play, The Velveteen Rabbit. She had a very large part and we were excited for her opening night. When the day arrived, I got up to care for mom and noticed that she was very lethargic. I called for the Doctor to come out and he said he would come by the next day. I had arranged for my friend Marsha, from church, to come and take care of mom while we were at the play. Marsha had been a nurse in the past and I fully trusted her to care for mom. When she came over, she took one look at my mom and said, "Je'net, it looks like your mom has turned a corner. I think we need to call the Doctor to talk about hospice. She really doesn't look good."

I had not realized it was that bad. I told her I would stay home and take care of her, but she said, "Look, Je'net, I can take care of your mom tonight. You need to be present for your family and your little ones. I doubt your mom is going anywhere tonight. I can wait for the Doctor. You won't get this night back with Jennifer. You need to go be there for her."

Reluctantly, I left with Pat, Jeremy, and Jennifer for the play. Jennifer was adorable and perfect. She even tossed us a wave from the stage when she was supposed to be pretending to be asleep and sick with scarlet fever. I am so glad I didn't miss that. At intermission, I called Marsha on the phone. She told me that when I got home, we would call a hospice company the Doctor had recommended and plan for some advanced care for mom.

When we returned that evening, all of us went in to see mom. Both the kids read to her from the Book of Psalms. Marsha told me that the Doctor said that mom could hang in for 6 days or 6 months. There was just no way to tell, but he did feel that we were at the end of our journey. I felt the need to call Chaplain Patricia Nesbit and pray over mom. Marsha headed home and promised to return in the morning. My husband and I held mom's hands and lifted her up in prayer while on the phone with the Chaplain that had led me to the Lord five years earlier.

In the middle of the prayer, mom gasped suddenly and then fell silent. It was as if she had waited for us to return to take her last breath. She passed on to heaven quickly surrounded by love with her family around her.

It is no small coincidence that she passed while we were together. Her passing could have come peacefully during any of the many moments that we were not by her bedside. This was God fulfilling a promise He had made to me that I would know when my mom passed and that she would be with angels.

My mom never called me by name in all the five years she lived with us. She didn't even respond to me calling her mom, only Dorothy. But one day, when I was tucking her into bed, I said as I did every night, "I love you, Dorothy."

She came into the room. She looked me in the eyes and said, lovingly, "I love you too, sweetheart."

All I ever wanted was for her to love me. And my prayers were answered.

Chapter 26
Finding My Purpose

My mother passed away in 2003. Finally, I felt that I had the freedom to pursue some work outside of the home. I had grown so much in my faith. I felt emotionally restored and physically ached to return to employment. With Jennifer in school at the Crystal Cathedral all day long, now I could manage a full-time job. I knew that I wanted to work in the non-profit sector. Having volunteered with the homeless and the incarcerated, I was hungry to make a difference.

I landed a job interview at Second Harvest Food Bank of Orange County. I was hired to coordinate special events and food drives. I was so excited to get a job at the same food bank that I had been getting food from for our homeless outreach. I knew several of the people who worked in the warehouse and the transition into this job was an easy one.

I could remember a time when I had paid for a motel room with the last change in my pockets and had not been able to buy Jeremy a 99-cent hamburger at the Carl's Jr. next door. We could smell the food cooking from the parking lot. I knew hunger in this personal way, not just for myself but as a parent who could not feed her children. This job really spoke to my heart.

In fact, we started our own little family project at home. Our family would shop and put together small food bags to drop off at local motels. The bags were intended to fill the gap for parents who had to choose between shelter and food as I had. Each bag had food that could be opened and eaten on its own or with just the use of a microwave. We made sure that we also included napkins and plastic forks or spoons so that whoever got the bag would feel the love we had for them and the respect we had for their dignity. We also gave bags like this out the window of our car at the freeway on and off ramps where the homeless would panhandle for food and money. I kept a cooler in my car so that I could offer an ice-cold beverage of water or soda to folks in need out in the hot sun. It was one thing to offer a bottle of water, but the expression of the recipient changed dramatically when their fingers touched the bottle and it was ice cold. They would raise their gaze just a little and look me in the eyes as if they were acknowledging that I truly saw them and their plight. I did.

It was easy to get behind this important cause. I particularly loved going to businesses that were hosting food drives and sharing in an impactful way how hunger was affecting our community. So many people in Orange County were surprised at the numbers and the stories that I presented. My stage experience supported my new public speaking responsibilities. I felt comfortable engaging groups with passion and earnest concern for those that went hungry in our own backyard. I believed now that God had given me those talents for this purpose. I was especially energized about the National Food Drive campaigns we participated in, like the "Stamp Out Hunger" postal workers food drive and the Scouting for Food with the Boy/Girl Scouts.

I stayed at this job for two years, but the tasks were limited and repetitive. I began to hunger for some more responsibility, perhaps in the area of fundraising or program development. I put out my resume and soon I was offered a job as a Development Associate at Giving Children Hope, a Christian organization that specialized in international relief work. I had just returned from a mission trip with my church to Uganda, where I was deeply affected by the depths of poverty that I witnessed there. Also, I was incredibly moved by the unshakable faith that the people of Uganda exhibited. The way they held up their love for Jesus was something to behold. It was humbling.

Jeremy had just graduated High School. I took him with me on that trip to Uganda. One day when we were setting up for our outreach activities,

Jeremy played his bagpipes as a way of announcing that the outreach was to begin. He was like a pied piper playing this strange sounding instrument that no one had ever heard before. The curiosity of the Ugandan people was overwhelming. We were overrun with children running out of the fields and into the area where we had set up our tent. We were worried we would not have enough supplies, but God had planned for this and we had literally just enough for the whole group.

My position at Giving Children Hope (GCH) was to help cultivate smaller donors, write grants and coordinate services as needed for the Executive Director. I enjoyed my job there. I was very blessed to travel to Liberia with the Williams Family, Jana and Todd, and their young daughter. The family had come to GCH needing our help in sending a container of goods to an impoverished country that borders Sierra Leone. Sierra Leone was in the news a lot at that time due to the blood diamond mines and child soldiers that were used as slaves by the RUF, Revolutionary United Front. The Williams partnered with the assistance of GCH to manage their family's dream to send school supplies to the children there. I helped Jana Williams in locating the supplies that they needed and arranging their trip. They surprised me with an offer to accompany them on their trip.

I have memories of joyful church services to tense moments on the border with some serious possible consequences. Vivid memories of this trip will stay with me forever! The village we traveled to had fresh bullet holes in all the buildings and community relations were complex and could change at any moment. Yet, our focus was on the children, and we felt assured that God had planned this trip and that He would keep us safe. Our accommodations were filled with love, but little else. There were showers, but the water didn't run, so we would pour cold water from a large trash barrel over our heads. It smelled like gasoline. The bathroom also came with its own *tarantula.* After the first couple of days, we just eyeballed one another from our separate corners of the room.

One night I awoke to the sound of scattering critters and let out a yelp as I they were crawling on my bed. One of the house helpers came running. I was horrified to see her stomp on the bugs and spiders with her bare feet. She just laughed at me and carried on. I remember how delighted I was when I used the bathroom on the plane coming home and the water was hot! What a luxury!

Back safe and sound in the United States, I took inventory of all that we had. Now that mom was gone, we had a spare room. It wasn't long before that empty bed got to me. There were still so many homeless on the streets and in the parks and riverbeds. I had met an older woman at a bus stop named Harriet and befriended her. She started to come to our monthly outreach at the church and it was obvious that she was struggling. She was 73, very tall with long silver hair. She walked with a cane and her legs were swollen and red. She had lost her home when her husband passed away. Harriet had been living on the top floor of a furniture store where someone had allowed her to store her belongings. She slept on her old bed with dressers and other furniture piled up all around her. It was a dangerous situation for her to get around in this makeshift attic apartment considering her mobility challenges.

Remarkable that the management had allowed it, but Harriet was paying them under the table from her limited social security. The new owner did not realize that she lived on the top floor. When Harriet asked if she could move a few things around to make it easier on her the new owner became understandably alarmed. Harriet was given 72 hours to vacate. Out of necessity, she began sleeping in her beat-up old Chevrolet. As a favor they gave her 6 months to find a new home for her belongings. After 6 months she was told they would remove and donate everything to Goodwill.

Harriet shared this story with me at one of our monthly events. Patrick and I decided that we could have her stay in mom's old room while we helped her look for a new apartment. She had the income from Social Security, so we just had to help her connect with something she could afford. This proved harder than expected as Harriet had very particular taste. She wasn't willing to move into the first several places we introduced her to.

I thought her reluctance to move to her own place was because she enjoyed our company and loved to tell us stories about her earlicr days as a writer in the film industry! She still wrote poetry and enjoyed sharing this as well. Eventually, we found a senior apartment complex that passed Harriet's stringent checklist. We helped her move her many, and I mean many belongings into her new place. For years we continued to visit Harriet at that apartment, and it warmed my heart to see her in her own kitchen.

After Harriet moved out, we helped another family. We helped a mom with three children who had been living in a camper until the father got arrested and the camper was impounded. Then we helped another single woman who I met at the Santa Ana Civic Center. Also, we helped a runaway teenager. One day my husband and I looked around and there were more people living with us than our little nuclear family.

I smiled and said, "Don't you think it's about time we got out of the way?"

And so, Grandma's House of Hope was born. In honor of the journey we had been on with my mother, we continued to call her old room, "Grandma's Room." We did some remodeling to add 2 additional bedrooms on to the house. In the middle of 2004, we opened the house as a women's transitional living home.

Over the next three years, I would learn as much about what I didn't want to do, as what I did. I wanted the women to have more support than a typical sober life provided. I added a food pantry and found someone to help out with job readiness. I had people offer to bring bible studies and 12 Step meetings to the house. I would celebrate holidays with small gifts and parties and always made it a point to learn everyone's name.

We funded the house by charging a program fee on a sliding scale but struggled to keep the beds full for a while. We allowed the women to come in without the ability to pay and then pay back the program fee when they became employed. But many of the women would come in for free, get a job, and then leave so they didn't have to pay back the amount we had temporarily sponsored them for. I felt we needed to add to the services we were offering. We had better retention after we offered case management, deliberate workforce development, and counseling.

To this day I continue to be grateful for our partnership with the Institute for Advanced Studies. They have generously provided therapists and supervision for little to no cost. We finally saw a small profit over our expenses as women were staying on and inviting friends to come too. We decided to file as a non-profit so that we could reinvest the excess income and further support the program.

Things were not always easy. There were phone calls in the middle of the night. Girls would sneak in a boy or get high. I understood why they pushed boundaries. Many of them were not ready yet to accept the help we were offering.

I stood in the front yard on a particularly challenging day. I was miserable after informing one of the ladies, Sarah, that she had to leave. I had discovered that she allowed her boyfriend to sneak into the house at night. This young girl at 22 years-old had arrived pregnant. She struggled to detox off heroin. 6 months later she gave birth to a healthy beautiful baby girl and had been doing a great job taking on motherhood. In fact, I had put her in charge as my house manager. But her boyfriend who had been incarcerated for the past year had gotten out of prison and come back into her life. He was not a positive influence and she was using again. I had to call for social services when she left the baby alone without supervision. She ran before they could get there.

I looked upward and asked God to make sense of this for me. Of course, he didn't answer that. Sarah was on her own journey and I had played my part. But I kept hearing him say this, "Where are you Je'net?"

I asked, "What Lord?" I didn't understand this at all.

"Where are you?"

It wasn't as if I heard something audibly, but the question kept incessantly crossing my mind. Perplexed I looked around me. The only thing that came to me was logical answers such as, "Well, Lord, I am on Paloma Ave."

I felt a Holy Spirit chill come over me. This was years after we had named our charity Grandma's House of Hope and designed our logo. The logo depicts a heart with a dove flying over it that represented the Holy Spirit. I stood in awe as I realized for the first time that the word, "Paloma" meant dove in Spanish. Further, "Oma" was the German word for grandma, and my husband's heritage was German. Could it be that God had this plan for me all along, and He was reminding me that He was in control?

But He wasn't done nudging me yet. The words, "Where are you" persisted. As I looked up and down the street, I realized one more thing. The cross street at the corner was named New Hope.

Grandma's House of Hope!

I could almost see Jesus standing in the middle of the street waving his arms.

My purpose for His kingdom was a long time in the planning. Long before I was even born, these streets had been named eternally for His purpose. Nothing random here.

Chapter 27
Fostering Hope

In 2007 I applied to work at the Orange County Rescue Mission. They were just opening the new Village of Hope and I was honored to be hired as a case manager for women and children. It was a long process to get hired, and I finally began work in early 2008, several months before the Village opened.

I loved working directly with women and kids. Particularly, one young woman made her way into my heart. Her name was Vivian and she was 18 years old. She had a rough time in her earlier years mostly fending for herself. Her mom was unstable, and Vivian had been left on her own many times growing up. She was Vietnamese and Chinese and a real beauty. More importantly, she was smart and a survivor.

She had a rough time at the Village. At 18 years old she was considered an adult in the program, but she still had a full year of High School to complete. She was dedicated to her studies and making good grades so that she could attend college. But her case at the Village was one of a kind. She had permission to leave the property every day on her bike and go to school. The policy at the Village was that no one could leave for the first 90 days for any reason. But they made an exception for Vivian. Yet, this put her at odds with the other women in the program so Vivian had a hard time making friends.

She loved to come into my office and talk to me. We spent time setting goals, but I also was an ear for her feelings of isolation. She shared with me about some of the trauma she had experienced living from home to home, sometimes with nowhere to sleep at night. Somehow, she had sidestepped foster services and made it work on her own. She took to calling me "Mama Je'net." When she would see me arrive at work, she would run across the yard and into my arms for a hug.

I learned a lot while working at the Village. But I was also laying the foundation for our first year at Grandma's House as a non-profit. I was developing my own policies and procedures, understanding bylaws and articles of incorporation, and recruiting my board of directors. Some of my founding members were Donna Schuller of the Crystal Cathedral, Susan Sherbert an author and expert in marketing, Nancy Watilo my daughter Jennifer's piano teacher, and Richard Henry from Wells Fargo Bank. My husband and I also served on the board.

We had received our first two foundation grants in 2007. One from Wells Fargo Foundation and another from the Klein Family Foundation. Each grant received was for our Nana's Kidz program, which focused on feeding hungry children living in motels in Orange County. The program fees received from our housing program were paid either by program participants or others on their behalf. Plus, the small individual contributions made up our funding model.

In 2007, Grandma's House of Hope joined the Orange County Human Trafficking Task Force and have been caring for survivors of sex trafficking and domestic servitude ever since. The task force was created and led by Community Service Programs (CSP). Recently this partnership with CSP was renamed, "Waymakers." The partnership would be a lasting one. We provided shelter for 2 survivors in 2008. They were brought to the United States from China and Ethiopia through an international trafficking ring. Ten years later we sheltered more than 45 survivors a year, and almost all of them were trafficked domestically within the US. Orange County, originally a pass-through county from San Diego to Los Angeles, had become a major destination for traffickers because of all the tourism and convention centers.

Most of the women who came to us had been lured into this way of life as young as 12 to 14 years old. Many were foster kids, or kids running away from abusive biological families. Hungry and with nowhere to sleep they had been befriended by someone who offered them basic needs like a hot meal or a warm coat. The kids were easy to spot for a trafficker. For instance, if an older man could approach a teenager in a mall and they were not immediately spooked, that would tell the perpetrator that she already had a familiarity with older men. Usually, the familiarity was because some abuse had already happened that had prompted them to run. It was enough to start a conversation that lead to dependence and then control. They were old beyond their years and severely traumatized by the time they were rescued and brought to us. I have been honored to have a seat on the Anti-Human Trafficking Congressional Advisory Committee led valiantly by Representative Ed Royce.

While going through the time-consuming process to settle our first survivor into our program, I realized it was time to renew our grant with the Klein Family Foundation. To my dismay, I had already missed the deadline! New to grant writing, I did not understand that I needed to submit a new Letter of Interest every year to gain permission to write the full application. There is usually no grace for this kind of mistake. In grant writing deadlines were deadlines. Sometimes a page out of order is enough to make a grantor set the application aside. Understandable given the number of applications for every grant dollar available.

I was beside myself! I really needed this $10,000 grant! I called the grants manager at the foundation and basically threw myself at her feet and begged for a second chance. The woman who answered the phone heard me out compassionately but held firm on the deadline. She declined my request for a time extension. She must have felt very bad for me because she did offer me the opportunity to write a letter to the Board Chair of the foundation. She said she would personally get the letter in front of her. I wrote a very heartfelt letter and hoped for the best. I knew I was learning a very painful lesson.

Not long after, I received a call from Catherine Sorensen, the acting Chair. She had read my letter. Although she did not have good news for me on the grant submission, she said she would like to meet me. I offered to give her a tour of our shelter and we set a time and date the following week. She drove out to the home in Garden Grove with her husband, Stan, who rested in the car while I walked her around.

Catherine was gracious and a great listener. After the tour we settled down for a glass of lemonade. After checking on Stan and giving him a glass of lemonade too, she asked me a lot of questions about how I got started and why. This was my first official site visit with a donor, and I was a bundle of nerves, but she put me at ease almost instantly. I felt free to share my vision, my story, and my commitment to helping the homeless. I thanked her for taking the time to come out and meet me and the ladies. Secretly, I held out some hope that she would tell me that we could still apply for that year's grant.

She didn't. She shared much better news with me. She told me that while the grant was off the table, she and the other board members each had some discretionary funds that they could award. Standing in the driveway she promised me that she would make Grandma's House of Hope one of the beneficiaries of this funding. She said she thought she could probably come up with around $25,000 to $30,000. I was in shock! I never imagined she would offer to give such an incredible gift to us. I was so grateful. In the end, when the check was finally written, Catherine gave GHH $80,000 that year!!! It was enough to open our second shelter, a 5-unit property where we could help 26 more women in need.

Catherine's generosity to Grandma's House of Hope has continued over the years. She is an amazing and courageous woman who I hold in the highest respect. She doesn't like to be publicly acknowledged because she has such a humble heart. So, I won't share any more details, but I will share that she is personally responsible for much of our continued growth. In 2015, I was honored to be part of a group who nominated her for the Association of Fundraising Professionals "Philanthropist of the Year" award on National Philanthropy Day. Seeing her get that award was especially rewarding for me and for the whole team at Grandma's House of Hope.

By February of 2009, I had made the decision to give up my job at the Rescue Mission and devote all my attention to growing Grandma's House of Hope. I rented a small office in a church in Garden Grove, built a tough shed in the parking lot to store our supplies for the Nana's Kidz program, and hired my first assistant, Lori Solomon. I also recruited a wonderful man named Saleem Majid to put together my books and file our first 990 tax return for 2007. I literally handed him a shoebox of receipts! He has supported the organization ever since. He is one of the most ethical, peaceful and honorable men I have ever known. The expenses that year came to a total of $26,000. The following year we would cross over $100,000. Within 10 years we had grown to an annual budget of over 3 million and growing. Such favor could only come by the hand of God.

I called my husband the day I resigned at the Mission and he supported my decision. He was out of town working in San Diego that week. As I recited off my plans for the near future, I casually added, "Oh, and Thursday we have to come by the rescue mission and pick up Vivian." There was a pause on the phone. Had I forgotten to mention that I wanted to offer Vivian a home with us to finish out her senior year in High School? Patrick was his usual easy going self and said, "Well, okay. Didn't know that was coming but we do have an extra bedroom, so okay let's do it!"

Vivian joined our family the following week. Although she currently lives with her Aunt Mary, she remains a part of our family to this day. She is at every holiday meal and birthday celebration and travels with us on family holidays. She is a very grown-up young lady now and I am very proud of her.

Pat and I enjoyed becoming a host family for Vivian. Later when Patrick retired, we would take this to the next level. In 2014, we decided to become foster parents. Our heart was the same as it is for the homeless that we serve. We wanted to help the kids that were difficult to place so we went into it thinking we would take in older kids and sibling sets or maybe pregnant teens. When we finished our 6 months of training, we were recruited for a special program for the county. Treatment Foster Care Oregon. TFCO is a wrap-around program for significantly challenged or traumatized youth 12 to 17 years old. The program is based in positive reinforcement for both the child and the family they have identified to return to. Both child and parents get an incredible amount of support through an extensive wrap-team including youth partners, Court Appointed Special Advocates, therapists, psychiatrists, and social workers. The child earns points every day to gain privileges the following week. As foster parents, we track 38 behaviors daily and call them in daily with 24/7 support. The child can never be left alone so they go everywhere with one of us, except when they are in school or with one of the team. Every week the foster parents meet for a two-hour case management meeting to discuss our children.

This is very rewarding, but a very difficult ministry at times. Our kids have had such trauma, they are very unpredictable and at times, even dangerous. There are only about ten families that are engaged in this program and the burn out can be significant. Some foster parents have been physically attacked by their kids or have had significant property damage as the kids work out their rage over their past. One of our kids tried to set her bedroom on fire, and another, just 14, ran away so many times that the police stopped coming by to make a report. But underneath all this behavior is just hurt and traumatized children who never got a chance at a supportive loving childhood. One of our kids experienced the death of his mother while in our care at the hands of her boyfriend. One of the most rewarding days I have ever had was watching this same boy reunite with a healthy family. He walked away from us after his

High School graduation, holding one sister's hand and carrying the other sister on his shoulders.

If every family would just carry one child on their shoulders, we could eliminate the foster care system and give these kids a fighting chance.

Chapter 28

God is Good, All the Time

Since we first began our ministry God has moved in such powerful ways. Like the Prayer of Jabez, He has expanded our territories.

In 2004, Grandma's House had one women's home with 10 beds, and we were supporting 10 children at a local motel with our Nana's Kidz program. Since then we have expanded to 14 shelter sites with a total of 157 beds that nightly bring warmth and comfort to the homeless. We have included 3 men's homes with our Grandpa's House program. In the last 15 years, we have rescued and restored over 2,300 of our county's most vulnerable and underprivileged.

And it all started with one person, reaching out to help one other person in need.

With God's favor, we now provide over 2.3 million meals to children and families who are unstably housed through our Nana's Kidz program. We opened a community center called Hope Works! We operate an Education and Enrichment Center for 45 families who live in a Section 8 low-income housing project. 16 of these families now have first generation college students! We have a donation center called, "Grandma's Attic" to respond to the generous contributions from our community.

Our mission remains to Empower the Invisible, those persons who are typically not eligible for, or have difficulty accessing other programs because of the complexity of their situations. Our mission is to minister to women and men who have faced trauma, victims of violent crimes or who are struggling with disabilities that make it difficult for them to quickly be housed. While the average stay in our program is 5 to 7 months, we do not have an arbitrary termination date for our services. It has been our mission to be the last program that someone needs, not just one of many.

To highlight a great program, our Healing House arose out of a need for safe and stable housing for homeless women who have been diagnosed with cancer or other chronic and serious illnesses. Homeless women who receive a diagnosis of cancer are typically looking at a difficult road to healing. Generally, they have not had access to preventative healthcare. In most cases, by the time they know they have cancer they are already at stage 3 or stage 4. Moreover, many hospitals will not offer chemo, radiation or other life-saving treatments if someone admits to being homeless. Grandma's House has walked with these women through recovery, remission, and through hospice. We are dedicated to caring compassionately for our ladies as they transition into the loving arms of Jesus. We continue to serve in memory of Marta, Eleanor, Dena, Debbie, Kathy, Renata, Abe and Loretta.

In 2012, Grandma's House started to work with the Orange County Healthcare Agency to provide housing and support for homeless persons with significant and persistent mental illness, substance use disorders, and formerly incarcerated individuals. In 2015, we received our first contract with CalOES (California Office of Emergency Services) to support our emergency shelter for victims of violent crimes. These last two relationships allowed us to make all our emergency services free to clients so they could save their money for permanent housing and a safe return to family and friends. We provide trauma-informed care to all our program participants. We recognize each one of them as individuals with stories that are unique and valuable.

Grandma's House of Hope filed its first financials in 2007. We raised just $26,000 that year and were a completely volunteer-run organization. Our budget in 2019 stands at $4,800,000. We currently support 38 staff members, 40% of whom have been homeless at some time in their lives. Several of our past program participants have gone to college to obtain their degrees in Human

Services and are now on staff and/or serving on our Board of Directors. Through outreach, prevention, shelter, and ministry, Grandma's House has touched the lives of over 23,000 people. To each of the 23,000, we offered love, hope, healing, and the promise of a forever home.

God is good, all the time. All the time, God is good.

Chapter 29
A Prayer for His Children

You are one person. You are flawed, imperfect, damaged, a sinner - a cracked vessel. But you are not an accident. You are not insignificant. You are worthy. You are a one of a kind unique masterpiece empowered by a God who intentionally gifted you for His purpose. You will stumble that is certain, but God will not allow a burden on you greater than what He puts within you to overcome it. He doesn't permit temptation that you cannot resist. In fact, temptations keep us dependent on God. Expect Him to help you. He will not disappoint. God is never late. God's grace is sufficient, and His power is made perfect in your weakness.

Whatever you have done, God forgives you. You are a work in progress. Always, God loves to use imperfect ordinary people to do extraordinary things. Forgive yourself long enough to lend a helping hand.

Suffering may be required to change what needs to be changed in your life, your family or your heart. But be encouraged! God uses problems to draw you closer. We pray our most authentic honest prayers when we are in pain. Thank God that he trusts you with this trial! He has a greater purpose for you on the other side of it.

Indeed, without God, life has no purpose. Without purpose, life has no meaning. Without meaning, there is no hope. When life has a purpose, you can bear almost anything.

You are as close to God as you choose to be, so choose to intentionally seek His friendship and let your worship be genuine and heartfelt. Live in peace with one another. Love should be your primary objective and greatest ambition. Life without love is worthless.

Treat this world as a temporary assignment and serve faithfully. Decide to grow and make an effort to do so. Be persistent! Experience life with others, share true feelings, encourage one another, support one another, and especially forgive one another. Speak the truth in love. Respect each other's differences and resist the temptation to gossip.

Remind yourself at the beginning of every day that you have a servant's heart. Think more about others than yourself. Attitude counts more than achievements. It's more important why you do something than what you do. Start with helping just one person without expecting a thank you.

You are a child of God, a new creation in Christ. Share this message.

Be God's messenger.

God wants to speak to the world through you.

About The Author

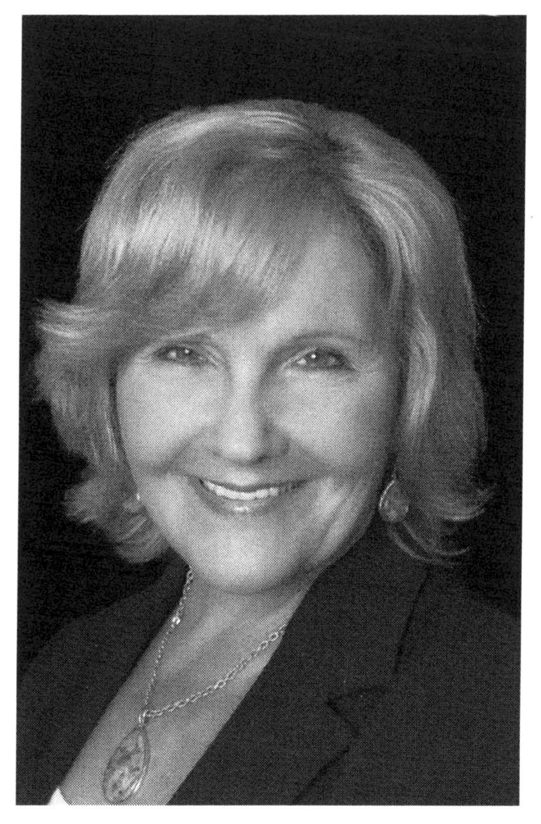

Je'net Kreitner is the founder of Grandma's House of Hope as well as several other incredible outreach programs. She has overcome many trials that have helped her grow and fueled her desire to help others.

Je'net is a great example of turning life's harshest lessons into life's greatest blessings.

After repressed memories of childhood sexual abuse surfaced in her mid 30's, Je'net experienced a series of unfortunate and catastrophic events, including a relationship with a controlling man that ended badly. Je'net found herself living homeless in California, with a young son to take care of. After hopeless months of struggling to survive on the streets and bouncing from one motel to another, an angel entered her life. A man she had met briefly saw something in Je'net as he visited with her, a goodness and potential that many overlooked because of her circumstances. After visiting with her only once, he offered to take both her and her son into his home. His faith in her and the unconditional help he offered them allowed Je'net to land back on her feet, and eventually he became her husband. Today, Je'net wants her programs to offer others the help and hope that she once so desperately lacked in her life. The support that allowed her to overcome immense trials and realize her amazing potential.

Je'net began her incredible journey to pay it forward at a monthly Homeless Outreach offered at her church in Orange, California, as well as volunteering with the Gleaners Jail Ministry Program. But after the death of her mother she wanted to do more and began by taking a woman into her home that she had befriended at a bus stop. The woman lived with Je'net and her family for a few months until they were able to find an apartment and help her get back on her feet. After that, the guest room in their home was constantly occupied with people who Je'net wanted to help. One day her husband remarked that there were more of these "guests" living in their house than family members. So, Je'net did the only thing that seemed to make sense, she, her husband, and her son moved out of the house and turned it into the very first shelter in 2004!

It was then that Grandma's House of Hope was founded as an effort to give back to a community that aided her in rebuilding her life after she was homeless in 1991. The purpose of Grandma's House is to Empower the Invisible, help women (and recently men, with the opening of Grandpa's House) to recover, heal and move forward in their lives. In addition to Grandma's House, Je'net also founded a Healing House program for homeless women with cancer. Providing a home to these women allows them to receive life saving chemotherapy and radiation treatments that are unavailable to those that cannot provide a house address, or other proof that they are not homeless. Other programs under Grandma's House include a Domestic Violence/Human Trafficking shelter, housing for women with Significant, Persistent Mental Illness, and Seniors with Disabilities who are unable to work. In 2007, Grandma's House of Hope officially became a nonprofit organization.

Je'net did not stop with just helping adults. Inspired by the haunting memory of her own child's hunger when they were homeless, Je'net created the Nana's Kidz Program. This weekend food program provides meals to children living in motels or doubled and tripled up with other families when the free meals at school are unavailable. She also started the HopeWorks! Education and Enrichment Center which is an after-school program for high risk kids in low-income neighborhoods. This program keeps children off the streets and out of gangs.. Through these programs, Grandma's House has rescued and restored over 2,500 women and men from homelessness, served over 2.4 million meals to the hungry, and provided outreach and referrals to over 26,000 families.

Today Je'net is considered a hero by the thousands of people whose lives she has blessed and is honored for her wonderful work. Rightfully so, Je'net was named Founder of the Year in 2014 for the Association of Fundraising Professionals' National Philanthropy Day and has been recognized as one of Orange County's 100 Most Influential People. She has also been recognized by the OC United Nations-Women's Division, multiple Soroptimist Chapters and elected Officials. She served (2) two-year terms on the Anti-Human Trafficking Congressional Advisory Committee. She was recently the recipient of a prestigious award at the Spirit Summit in Los Angeles. She continues to spread her messages of hope and healing through speaking platforms. To learn more about Grandma's House of Hope please visit www.GrandmasHouseofHope.org or call 714.558.8600.